weaning
made simple

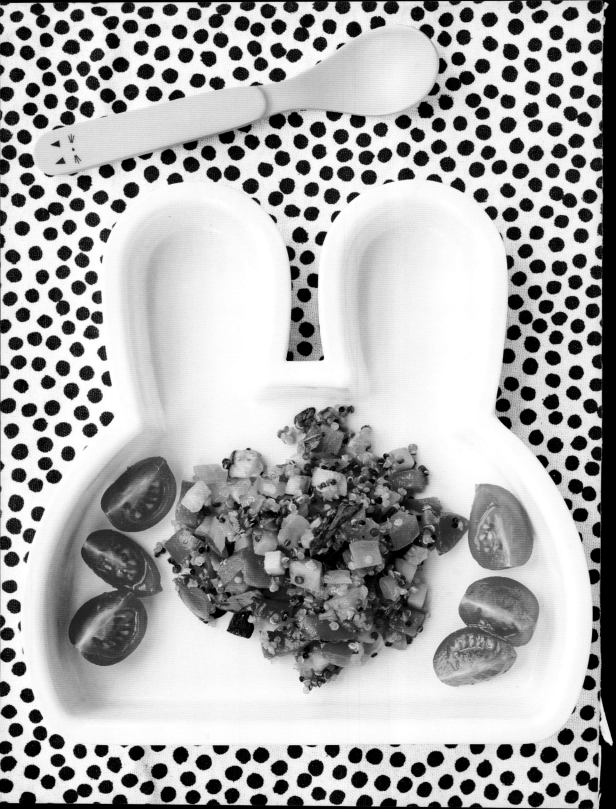

weaning made simple

Your go-to guide to baby's first foods

Annabel Karmel

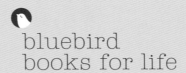

bluebird
books for life

First published 2020 by Bluebird
an imprint of Pan Macmillan
The Smithson, 6 Briset Street, London EC1M 5NR
Associated companies throughout the world www.panmacmillan.com

978-1-5098-9264-8
A CIP catalogue record for this book is available
from the British Library
Printed and bound in China

Publisher Carole Tonkinson
Managing Editor Martha Burley
Art Direction & Design Nic & Lou
Senior Production Controller Sarah Badhan
Prop Styling Charlie Phillips
Food Styling Lizzie Harris

Nutritional Consultant Rosan Meyer M. Nutr, PhD has worked closely with Annabel Karmel in
providing the correct introductory nutritional information and weaning guidance in this cookbook.

Visit www.panmacmillan.com to read more about all our books and to buy them. You will also find
features, author interviews and news of any author events, and you can sign up for e-newsletters so that
you're always first to hear about our new releases.

contents

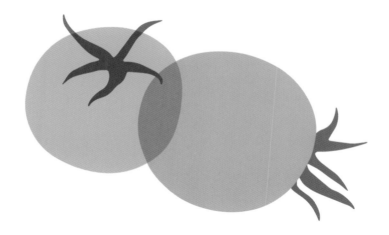

weaning made simple

How do I know my baby is ready for weaning? What should I be giving them? How much is too much or too little? What if they hate my cooking? What if they won't try new things? What if my baby chokes? What if they refuse food? Overwhelmed and under pressure. That's how countless parents feel when starting out on their baby's weaning journey. But it doesn't need to be complex!

As families hit this major milestone (and doesn't it creep up on us ever so quickly?), 'worry' often far outweighs the 'wonderment', and 'fear' overshadows the 'fun' that parents are expected to have when feeding. It's time to set expectations aside.

Weaning can be mighty challenging. Fact. There is no one-size-fits-all for getting your baby eating like a food pro. There is no step-by-step manual to producing the perfect eater. That would be far too easy. After all, we all know how parents love a challenge!

I wouldn't have spent my life's work helping families with advice, support and recipes if feeding baby was 'simple' and 'magical'. The intense pressure many parents feel to 'get it right' (and I've experienced this first-hand myself) can be all-consuming. Compounded by the fact that there is a world of conflicting information and advice out there, it's completely natural to feel defeated before you've even dabbled with those first foods.

You're probably wondering why my book is named *Weaning Made Simple*, when in actual fact, weaning can be fraught with complications.

Having spent over 27 years researching baby and child nutrition, developing recipes and providing practical support to weaning families, I know what babies need in order to lay the foundations for a lifetime of healthy eating. And this new book cuts through all the unnecessary jargon and outdated advice to provide exactly what you need to know and do.

No frills. Just the practical information and easy-to-follow guidance for getting your baby to a great place as they reach their first birthday. The reality is, your baby is not going to automatically like all the foods you want them to like. Weaning is about working through flavours and textures, helping them to enjoy the foods that meet their needs nutritionally.

Are you ready to join me? It's time to banish that build-up of worry and offload expectation. We're on this journey together, so relax, go at their pace and take it one meal at a time. Let's go!

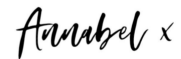

Annabel x

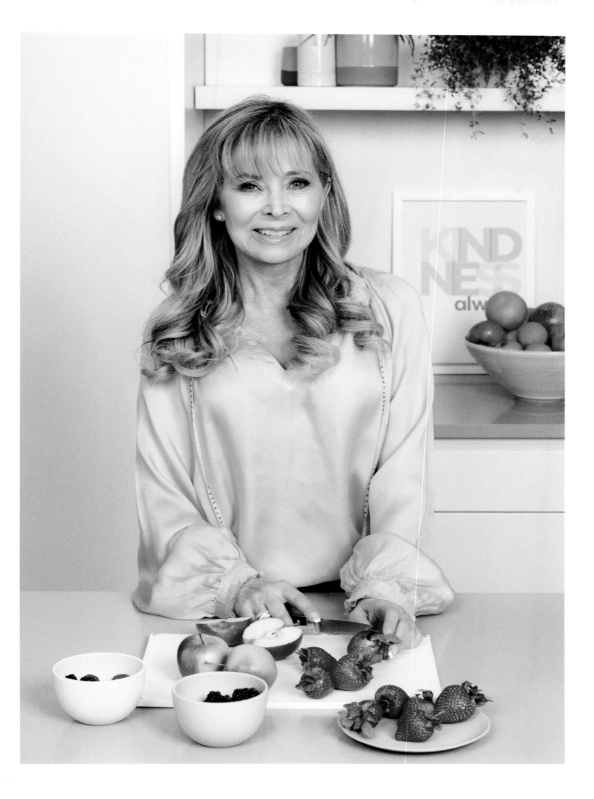

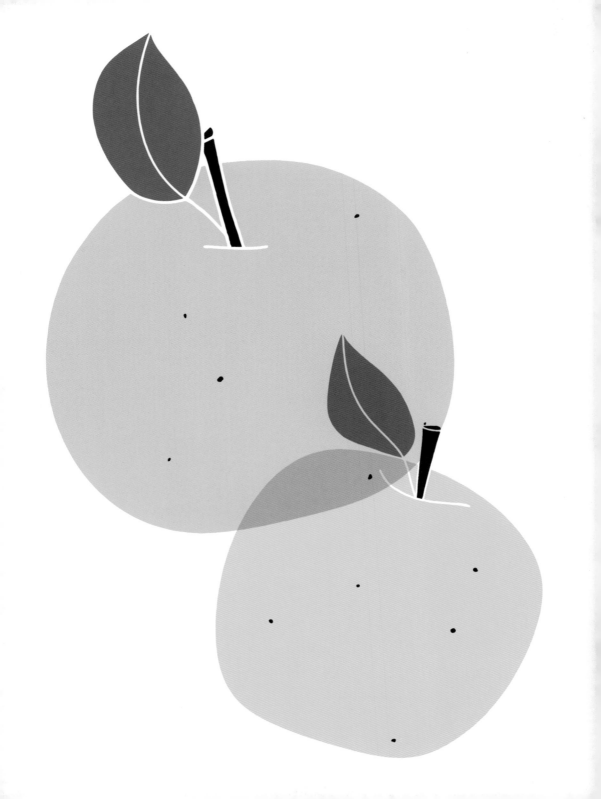

chapter 1

weaning basics

what is weaning?

We use the term weaning to mean moving your baby from milk to solid food. It is also talked about in terms of moving your baby from breast to bottle or even weaning your baby off a dummy, although in this book our focus is on solid food.

Weaning is a gradual, gentle process and one that is learned. Before babies learn to walk, they roll, crawl, stumble and fall. Yet, we keep encouraging them until they can walk unaided, and parents should take the same approach to introducing food.

Weaning is about introducing a variety of flavours, tastes and textures. It's about teaching her how to eat solid foods and explore a wide variety of nutritious foods that will provide a great foundation for her future health. The important thing is to start slowly, at a comfortable pace for your baby.

YOUR BABY'S USUAL MILK FEEDS

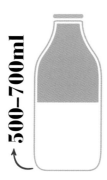

500–700ml

Weaning is a gentle process, so it's important to remember that your baby's usual milk will still remain the most essential dish on the menu with around 500–700ml of breast milk or formula needed each day up until her first birthday.

Up until your baby has reached 12 months, the aim during this time is to introduce a variety of foods to support your baby's growth and development, but it's important to note that she will still rely on breast or formula milk to offer a complete balance of nutrients needed at this crucial stage of development.

However, from around 6 months, your baby's regular milk will no longer provide her with all of the nutrients she needs – in particular iron (see page 40). Full term babies are born with reserves of key nutrients inherited from mum, but by 6 months, her stores of these start to deplete, which means that milk is no longer a one-stop shop for all-round nourishment. Instead, nutrient-rich foods need to be included in her diet to supplement her regular milk. We'll go on to talk about all those important nutrients including iron, essential fatty acids and protein-rich foods on pages 36–43.

Once your baby starts to move on to three meals at around 6 months, you can bring her milk feeds down to 3–4 milk feeds per day (total milk still around 500–700ml). Check out my meal planner on page 14 as a guide on how to combine milk feeds with mealtimes.

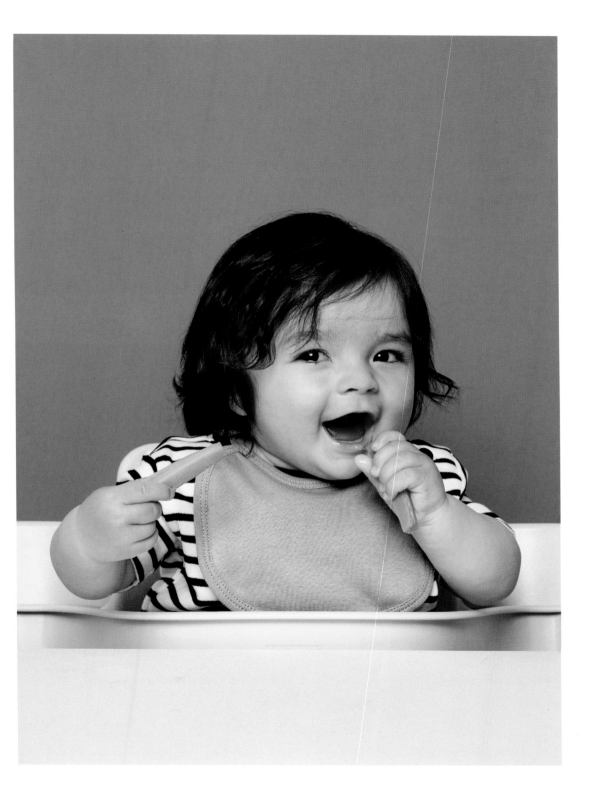

COMBINING MILK & SOLID FOODS

At this stage it's about introducing a variety of new tastes and textures rather than volume of foods that contribute nutrients and calories (not just yet anyway). If you're thinking of starting your little one on her weaning journey a little before 6 months (and we'll come on to this shortly) then remember that it is more about introducing new foods than giving a full meal. You'll need to build up to this gradually.

During those early stages of weaning, parents sometimes (and understandably) offer food when their babies are hungry, when in actual fact, they just need a milk feed. Introducing solids too early (under 4 months of age) may have a detrimental effect on the immature digestive system and could lead to anaemia by displacing their regular milk with vegetables and fruit, which are low in iron. When starting out weaning, it is best not to change your usual milk feeding pattern.

Around 6 months

What is the right amount to begin with? Start with food just once a day, around midday, and if she seems to enjoy it, you can gradually progress to two meals, and then three meals, until she's enjoying her breakfast, lunch and dinner just as you would. Every baby is different but most parents find it easiest to continue with the morning and evening feeds and fit the other milk feeds around baby's new mealtimes, gradually following the hunger and fullness cues giving a little less milk as their baby takes more solids. It's worth noting that during this time, with so many new and interesting foods to explore, she is likely to naturally have less of an appetite for milk.

To ensure they still get enough of the white stuff, formula or breast milk can be added to purées and will count towards her overall milk intake.

Drinking water

Introduce a cup from around 6 months and offer sips of water with meals. Using an open cup or a free-flow cup without a valve will help your baby learn to sip and is better for her teeth.

---

myth buster

I can't give my baby tap water

Tap water is perfectly fine for your baby from 6 months (so long as the supply is safe). It is only necessary to boil tap water to kill any bacteria if using with formula.

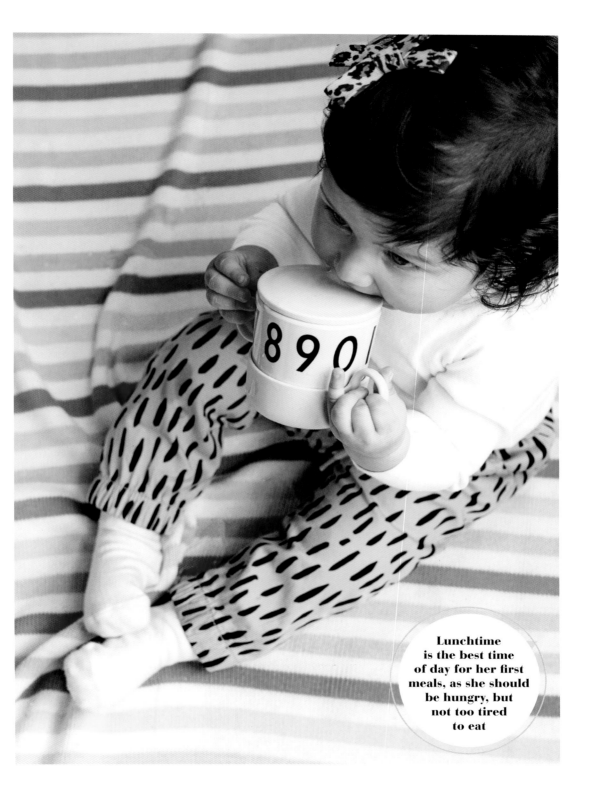

Lunchtime
is the best time
of day for her first
meals, as she should
be hungry, but
not too tired
to eat

HOW TO COMBINE SOLID FOODS WITH MILK FEEDS

This is intended as a reference to the first weeks of weaning, but always be guided by your baby's appetite: some will want to go faster, whereas others will take longer to move on. If you are starting a little before 6 months, only give your baby purées. You can introduce finger foods at 6 months. I will go on to explain more about this later.

	WEEK 1	WEEK 2 & 3	WEEK 4
Waking	Milk	Milk	Milk
Breakfast		Solid food (purée/finger food), **water** to drink	Solid food (purée/finger food), **water** to drink
Mid-morning	Milk	Milk	Milk
Lunch	Solid food (purée/finger food), **water** to drink	Solid food (purée/finger food), **water** to drink	Solid food (purée/finger food), **water** to drink
Mid-afternoon	Milk	Milk	Milk
Tea			Solid food (purée/finger food), **water** to drink
Bedtime	Milk	Milk	Milk

Breast milk and/or formula should still be given as your baby's main milk as cow's milk has a lower amount of many key nutrients, in particular iron. However, you can give small amounts of cow's milk with cereal or in cooking from 6 months. Stick to full fat milk (for example, if you're making cauliflower cheese) as the calories will help fuel your baby's growth.

➤ **By 7 months**, once first tastes have been established and your baby has started to explore finger foods, you should be aiming for around three small meals a day. Usually you will find that your baby will naturally show signs of wanting to reduce milk feeds and so you can bring these down to three to four feeds per day (total milk around 600ml). At this stage it is still common for many babies to wake at night for a milk feed. This is fine, but aim for no more than four milk feeds a day (over a 24 hour period) and ensure that they are taking sufficient solids and drinking water.

Most babies will naturally reduce the amount of milk they consume as they increase their food intake. However, some babies may need a helping hand to cut down in order to have any kind of incentive to try food. She will need to learn to recognise when she is hungry and full-up, and if she isn't reducing her milk intake, it could delay her progress with weaning.

➤ **By 10 months**, there are so many tasty new foods to try that your baby will be consuming slightly less milk and will have probably dropped another milk feed (total milk around 500ml per day) as she will now be having the likes of yoghurt and cheese in her diet too. Carry on reducing her milk feeds down to two to three feeds a day as you want her to be exploring as many different foods as possible. At this stage, finger foods, chopped foods or small portions of a suitable family meal (avoiding those foods listed on page 46) will take centre stage and purées should now be off the menu. You can also introduce a small mid-morning or -afternoon snack instead of one of her milk feeds.

➤ **By 12 months**, you can switch to full fat cow's milk as lots of important nutrient packed goodness will now be coming from food. Cow's milk is also an ideal source of bone-boosting calcium, as well as vitamin D, which helps the body take in all that calcium. If you are breastfeeding, then it is perfectly fine to continue doing so – the World Health Organisation advise continuing until your baby is 2 years old in addition to solid food. Just ensure that cow's milk or breastfeeds do not replace food, and that your toddler does not have more than 500ml of cow's milk per day as this can lead to iron deficiency and further feeding difficulties.

myth buster

I shouldn't offer cow's milk before 12 months

Cow's milk should not be consumed as a drink until 12 months, but you can use it from 6 months in recipes. So long as your baby is getting their recommended daily intake of breast milk or formula, then you can include cow's milk in your baby's cereal and recipes and cow's milk products like yoghurt and cheese.

WHEN TO INTRODUCE SOLIDS

Put simply – around 6 months of age. Of course, some babies will show signs of being ready before, but 'around 6 months' is the age advised by the World Health Organisation. Babies should never be weaned before 4 months (17 weeks) as their digestive systems aren't mature enough to cope with food at this point. So what are the signs that your baby is ready to take that leap?

SIGNS SHE'S READY

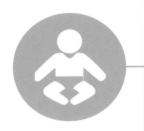

She is sitting up and supporting her own head
This doesn't have to mean sitting up completely unsupported, just as long as she can sit up for 3–5 seconds on her own. This is why a highchair will be your most important piece of weaning kit as it will provide that additional support for her feet, bottom and back while eating.

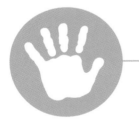

She has developed hand-to-eye coordination
She needs to be able to coordinate food and direct it into her mouth. Is she trying to stick her fingers, fists and everything in sight into her mouth? That is a good sign she's mastered this skill.

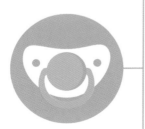

She is showing signs that she has lost an early baby reflex, called tongue-thrust
This is a protective reflex to help prevent babies from choking. As soon as something foreign is put on your young baby's tongue, the tongue-thrust reflex means she'll try to push it out of her mouth. This reflex is likely to have disappeared by 6 months, meaning she is better able to move food from the front to the back of her mouth and then swallow it. Not all babies lose this reflex by 6 months, but when weaning starts, it is likely this will soon disappear.

RED HERRINGS

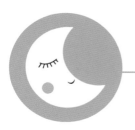

Waking more at night
There is no hard evidence to suggest that sleep is a factor affected by weaning. And it's a myth that full babies sleep through the night (sorry folks!). There are all sorts of reasons why your baby may be waking through the night. She may need a feed, she may want your comfort and reassurance during the night, or she may benefit from a more consistent bedtime routine to help her settle. Teething can also upset your baby's routine and sleep patterns.

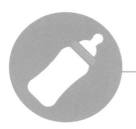

When she is still hungry after a milk feed
This is more likely to be down to a growth spurt. Learning a new skill requires additional energy. Sometimes this could be a mental development and you might not see any noticeable changes other than that she has an increased appetite because she needs fuel. Sometimes parents think their baby needs food but actually she needs more milk. Giving your baby food when she is not developmentally ready can lead to gastrointestinal problems and can also be linked to anaemia.

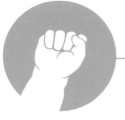

Fist chewing
This is a phase called mouthing and lots of babies tend to do this. Their mouths are highly sensitive and they learn through sensations in their mouths which helps prepare them for solid foods. This is why you will find her putting toys or fists into her mouth — to get that feedback from those sensations.

When she seems more interested in food
Babies are instinctively curious about the world around them and will naturally show signs of being interested in what you are eating. That doesn't mean they are necessarily ready for solids.

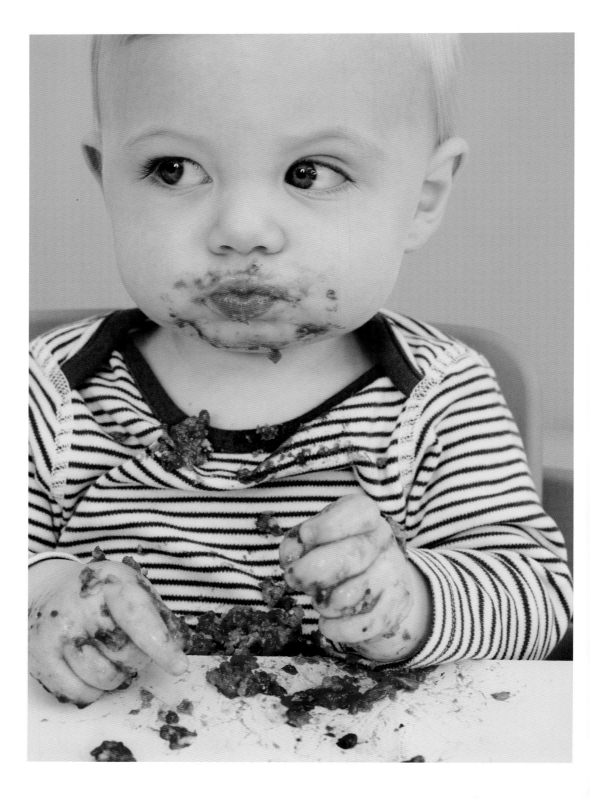

Bigger babies need to be weaned earlier

Babies who are big for their age do not need solids earlier than other babies. It's easy to see why people might think that, but remember, it's what's going on inside that counts. Babies are ready for solids when their digestive systems are developed enough to cope. That's not before 17 weeks (4 months). Speak to your health visitor if you are unsure.

Calming those jitters

The first time you feed your baby those first tastes, the chances are you'll be far more nervous than her.

She is experiencing new and exciting things every hour of the day, so it's likely she'll take this in her stride. And let's face it, she'll soon let you know if she's enjoying a new taste or wondering what on earth she's eating. Her initial responses are all part of the fun! Don't worry if she spits food out. It's all part of the learning process.

PREMATURE BABIES

Babies born before 37 weeks will have fewer nutritional stores than full-term babies and premature babies who are breastfed will require a multivitamin containing high levels of vitamin D and an iron supplement. Some mums may also be given a supply of breast milk fortifier to help enrich their breast milk. Bottle-fed premature babies will be given prescription milk that is higher in energy, protein and fortified with higher levels of vitamins and iron. A dietitian will be able to advise when to switch to regular formula, this will depend on how prematurely your baby was born.

If your baby was born prematurely, start weaning her between 4–6 months post term age. This is to ensure she is developmentally ready to digest solid foods, while at the same time balancing the need for more nutrients. As with all babies, check for the key signs she might be ready to start weaning (see page 16). Premature babies should be reviewed regularly by a registered dietitian who is qualified in children's nutrition.

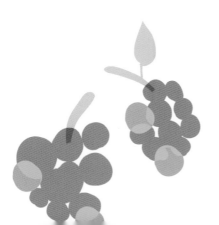

choosing the right approach for your baby

Traditional spoon-led or baby-led? It is completely up to you which method you choose to adopt and what works for your family. The important thing is that both you and your baby feel content and comfortable in your routine.

➤ **Spoon-led weaning** is often seen as a more gentle approach to weaning, as it is a gradual progression onto more textured solids. With this approach you will start with a smooth, slightly runny purée, which will be only ever so slightly thicker than the milk they have been used to, probably something like a runny yoghurt. You then steadily start to introduce thicker and more textured foods over the coming weeks and months.

Spoon-led weaning also allows you to take full control of exactly what and how much your baby is eating and allows you to monitor their nutrient intake more closely, which reassures many parents.

➤ **Baby-led weaning** has never been more popular. The theory is that you start with soft finger foods and small portions of family meals from six months. The idea behind it is that you take a step back and put your baby in control, allowing and encouraging them to go at their own pace while exploring a variety of foods, tastes and textures for themselves.

Baby-led weaning encourages hand-to-eye coordination and regularly handling foods improves their dexterity, which is a hugely important skill for your baby to master. With baby-led weaning your baby essentially eats what the rest of the family are eating (albeit suitably chopped or mashed to begin with) minus any added salt. This means that mealtimes become more of a social occasion because your baby is watching how the rest of the family are eating and essentially copying how it's done.

Plus, this also means less time spent preparing foods as your little one is eating what everyone else is having. And lots of families who adopt this approach find that their usual meals become healthier as they cater for baby too.

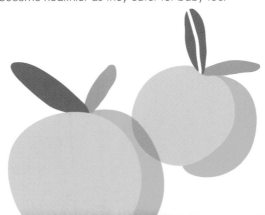

COMBINING PURÉES & FINGER FOODS

Both methods have their advantages and disadvantages but it really is a personal choice. While lots of parents have success with spoon-led or baby-led weaning alone, combining the two is most suited to lots of families.

Prior to 6 months, babies tend not to have developed the hand-to-eye coordination needed for baby-led weaning, so it's not an option if your baby is ready to wean early or for those babies who have a medical condition and have been advised to start a little earlier than 6 months. In this case, purées or well-mashed food are an obvious bridge between milk and solid foods.

Around 6 months, whether baby-led weaning or not, babies should be having soft finger foods, even if alongside mashed food or purées. And those babies who are baby-led weaning will still need to have smooth foods such as yoghurt to learn about these textures. Regularly offering a variety of family meals and finger foods encourages babies to adopt good eating habits from the very start as they get to experience a more varied range of tastes and textures than they might on a spoon-fed diet. That being said, there is no reason why you can't mash or purée certain family meals if they're not quite ready for baby-led weaning.

Giving purées when your baby is ready for first foods (particularly if slightly earlier than 6 months), with the introduction of finger foods and family meals from around 6 months is a fantastic flexible option. This is also advocated by the likes of the Department of Health, the NHS and the British Nutrition Foundation.

What's important is that there is no right or wrong to weaning. Some babies thrive on purées, others on finger foods and yet some on both. Instead of committing to a certain feeding method, it's OK to be flexible in your approach and to follow your intuition and your baby's developmental signs.

myth buster

Babies need to eat rather than play with their food

Embrace your baby's weaning journey and encourage playing and exploring with food's flavours and textures as much as possible. After all, taste is just one of the five senses. Get the most out of each meal time by offering a finger food along with a dip or purée for a hands-on weaning experience.

getting started with first purées

Weaning is a slow and steady process, and when you know your baby is ready for solids, a few tastes are likely to be sufficient at first. If you're starting a little before 6 months, explore fruit and vegetables first before introducing other foods from around 6 months of age.

FIRST TASTES

Babies are born with mature taste buds for sweet, bitter, sour and savoury tastes. However, they will be exposed to breast or formula milk first, which contains lactose, which is naturally sweet. They will therefore happily accept sweet foods.

Although their bitter and sour taste buds are mature at this age, as they have not been exposed to these tastes before, they will need to develop them through food exposure. It is absolutely fine to still offer sweet veg alongside but you just need to ensure you are also offering the bitter vegetables, such as spinach or broccoli, during those early days too.

Start with a single vegetable – sweet root vegetables are a great place to start such as sweet potato, carrot or butternut squash. You then also need to introduce those more bitter tastes such as cauliflower, spinach and broccoli sooner rather than later and repeat these tastes, as your baby will then be more receptive to new foods before she reaches 10 months. These vegetables can be boiled or steamed and blended to a purée – you want your purée to be very smooth, with no lumps – the consistency of runny yoghurt is a good guide to follow.

If you are starting at 6 months, it's important to introduce foods containing critical nutrients, like iron, fairly quickly. Offer fruit and veg for

---

myth buster

Avoid introducing meat and other protein

*Red meat, chicken and fish **should** be introduced to your baby from 6 months, and are an essential part of their diet, as they are iron rich. Make sure they are cooked thoroughly and check well for bones before offering to your baby. Lentils and pulses are also protein rich and make a great addition at this time, too.*

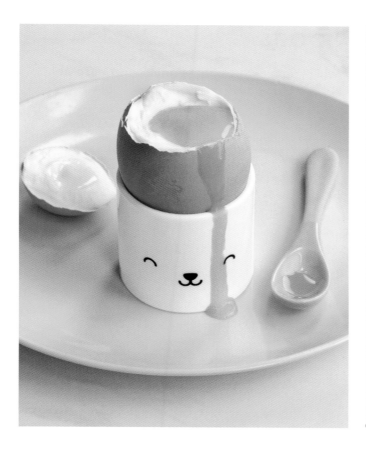

Runny eggs are back on the menu

Eggs are one of the most nutritious foods available and your baby can eat them runny when you start weaning at around 6 months following a Government change in advice in 2017, as long as they have the British Lion mark on. Eggs contain specific nutrients to support your baby's growth, including folate, vitamin D, iodine, selenium, choline and omega 3 fatty acids. Check out egginfo.co.uk for more information. But, it's safe to say you can go ahead and scramble, poach and boil away!

the first two weeks and then start introducing protein-rich foods like red meat and oily fish such as salmon.

Baby rice has historically been the first weaning food for many babies. However, questions have been raised with regard to its contribution towards a baby's nutrient intake, and also its arsenic content, which seems to be higher in rice-based porridges than other grain-based porridges. While there is no harm in giving baby rice and it can still form part of your baby's diet, it is good to introduce

other grains including millet, oats and quinoa to vary not only the taste exposure but expand nutrient intake.

From 6 months, you can also start to introduce soft finger foods like banana or ripe peach that can be 'gummed' to a suitable consistency. The more your baby experiments with finger foods the quicker she will become proficient at feeding herself.

OFFERING NEW FOODS

While each and every baby will progress through weaning at a different pace, here is a guide to the kinds of foods that are good for your baby's growth and development as they go through the stages.

AGE	FOODS	CONSISTENCY	ROUTINE
Between 4–6 months (if your baby is ready to start solids)	Start with 1–2 root vegetables and then add bitter tasting vegetables such as broccoli, spinach, or kale Offer a different vegetable each time as variety is key. By week 2, start to combine different flavours and introduce fruit Porridge	Thin, smooth purées	Start with one small food offering and then increase to two for weeks 2 and 3. By week 4, they should be on three small meals a day Give usual milk on demand
From 6 months	Fruit and vegetables Meat, poultry, fish, eggs, full fat milk products Grains (wheat, oat, quinoa) Full fat natural yoghurt	Thicker purées and mashed foods Well-cooked meat Soft finger foods	Limit purées and progress to offering three meals a day within two weeks – breakfast, lunch and dinner Include iron-rich foods and foods that contain essential fatty acids (see page 39) e.g. salmon Give usual milk, but do not replace mealtimes with milk

AGE	FOODS	CONSISTENCY	ROUTINE
From 8–10 months	Family foods (avoiding those listed on page 46) Start giving complete meals (e.g. Mini cottage pies, page 228) as well as separate finger foods Offer smaller finger foods so your baby can practise her pincer grip	Complete family meals chopped or mashed to the right consistency for baby Wider variety of finger foods, including smaller foods (e.g. pumpkin seeds, raisins	Continue to offer three meals per day and start to introduce a small healthy snack (mid-morning or mid-afternoon) instead of their usual milk, if your baby requires this **Note:** *this will depend on their milk feeds. If milk is cut out between breakfast and lunch for example they will need a snack, but if they are still having milk then, a snack is not needed*
From around 10 months	Fruit and vegetables Meat, poultry, fish, eggs, full fat milk products Grains (wheat, oat, quinoa) Full fat natural yoghurt	Complete family meals but start to mash and chop less Continue to offer a wide variety of finger foods	Continue to offer three meals per day, plus one or two healthy snacks (mid-morning or mid-afternoon), if needed – depending on your baby's requirements – instead of their usual milk

25

Snacks

Crafting healthy snacks can be another way of getting those all-important nutrients into your baby's diet. From 10 months, she can be having two small but nutritious snacks per day in between meals. Try to make sure that snacks contain at least two critical nutrient food items (see page 36), one of which could be her milk.

It is important to note that this is just a guide. We want baby to be hungry for their next main meal, and some babies will need smaller or fewer snacks than others.

When will they eat what we're eating?

They can eat what you're having, although foods may need to be adapted in texture (e.g. blended to varying degrees) and ingredients (e.g. no added salt or sugar). Get to know the foods to avoid before the age of 12 months (check out page 46 for my guide) and go and explore the world of food. A little tip: babies are great at mimicking your behaviour, so whenever you can, eat with them. They are not born knowing how to feed themselves, so encourage them to watch and copy you.

SNACKS FROM 10 MONTHS

Small cubes of cheese with cucumber sticks

Fresh fruit pieces and yoghurt

Carrot batons and hummus

Toasted pitta spread with cream cheese

Unsalted and unsweetened rice cakes and banana slices

Avocado slices and mini breadsticks

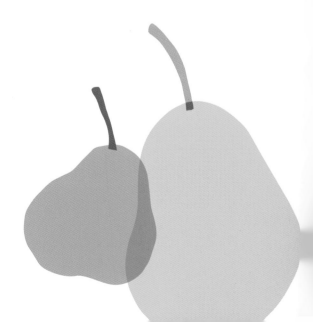

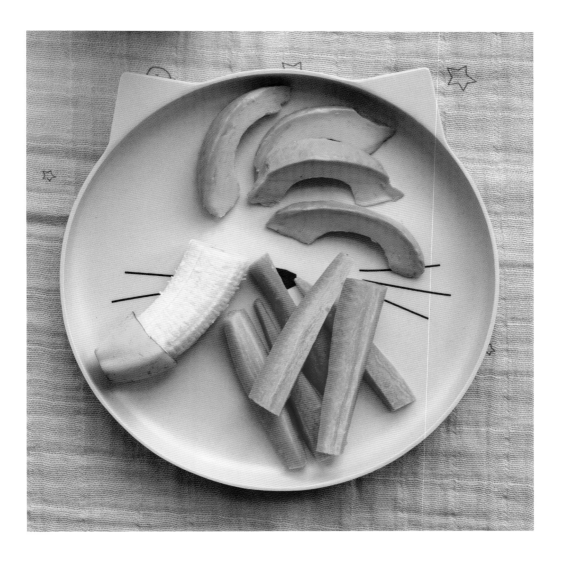

did you know?

Ripe fruit is important

Ripeness in fruit is an extremely important aspect to support digestion. Ripeness is all about texture and being able to physically manage eating the food. For example, a ripe banana is soft and squishy, and perfect for your baby. A ripe avocado is another of nature's natural convenience foods and they are full of goodness.

27

INTRODUCING NEW TEXTURES

Eating is a skill and tackling texture is another developmental milestone that they have to train for whilst on their weaning journey.

As well as learning about the different tastes on offer, different textures must also be introduced early on as there is evidence that those who wait until their baby is over 10 months are more likely to develop problems later as toddlers and become fussy eaters, simply because these skills haven't been learnt.

Babies don't need teeth to chew – their teeth are sitting under their gums, which are very hard and will be able to tackle all kinds of textures.

Whether you are going down the baby-led weaning route or adopting a more traditional spoon-led approach (see page 20), by around 6 months she should be on soft finger foods and mashed food (rather than finely blended purées). If you are baby-led weaning, you should still offer smooth foods such as yoghurt. Not only is this a great source of calcium, but this is still a different texture she needs to explore and accept.

PORTION SIZE

There are not set portion size guides for children under 12 months as every baby is different, so it is important to follow a responsive feeding approach which loosely means going at their own pace.

Start with just one meal a day and follow her lead. Don't expect her to take more than 1–2 teaspoons to begin with. If she seems keen and is taking more, then that's a bonus. If this is the case you can progress to two meals a day, and then be on three meals a day by 4 weeks. But remember, she'll set the pace.

TACKLING TEXTURE

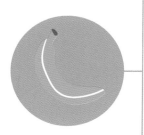

Gradually start to mash a bit of her favourite purée as a step on from blending the complete meal to a smooth consistency. Having a thicker purée with mashed up pieces leads her to adopt a more lateral tongue movement (which is another key learning step in mastering the art of eating), which also means less chance of gagging. Soft finger foods that will squash between your thumb and forefinger can be a great stepping stone to get your baby onto slightly lumpier foods. 'Bite and dissolve' finger foods or snacks are good, then she can progress to toast as this also dissolves but has a slightly trickier texture to manage.

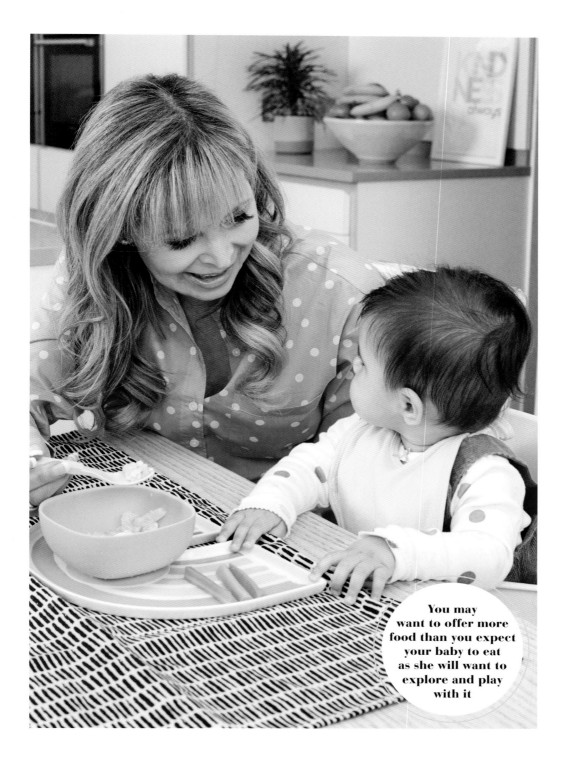

You may want to offer more food than you expect your baby to eat as she will want to explore and play with it

best first finger foods

From 6 months (whether or not you started to wean your baby earlier than the recommended time), you can introduce soft finger foods to your baby.

She will need to be able to close her hand around the food so it's best to start with pieces that are big enough for your baby to hold in their fist with some sticking out. Fairly long pieces (roughly 5–6cm) stand a better chance of being picked up.

When starting out with finger foods you should take the skin off most fruits and vegetables. The skin introduces a new texture, which can be difficult to manage and can lead to choking, and the fibre content is also quite high. From around 10 months of age, when she has got to grips with finger foods, you can keep skin on fruit/veg that has thin skin (e.g. nectarine, ripe pear, peach).

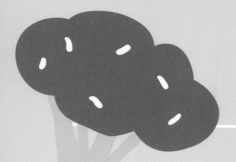

SOFT FRUIT AND VEG

Broccoli florets
Banana 'lollipops'
Mango slices
Avocado slices
Carrot batons
Butternut squash wedges

**Find out how
to prepare
on pages
76–89**

OTHER SOFT FOODS

Quartered cooked eggs
Pasteurised cheese
(such as mild cheddar or mozzarella)
Pieces of cooked fish
Pieces of cooked chicken
Wholegrain toast fingers

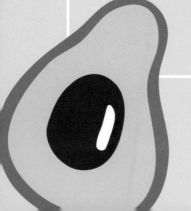

tips for happy weaning

It might seem as easy as 1, 2, 3 to us, but mastering the art of eating requires a lot of concentration, practice (and patience) for baby. It's a skill she has to learn in the same way that she would to roll, crawl and talk. And it's a tricky one as foods come in all shapes, sizes and consistencies, let alone colours and flavours. It must be pretty mind-blowing for a baby!

To give her a helping hand in mastering this new skill, you need to try and ensure that her total concentration is focused on the food in her mouth. Most importantly, ensure that she is stable and secure so that her undivided attention is on her food rather than trying to keep herself steady and comfortable.

It's all in the timing

It is entirely up to you as to when you decide to get started weaning as it will be a case of fitting in with your family's routines. However, you might find it useful to consider the following:

> **WHEN SHE IS MOST ALERT** – perhaps after a nap and not directly before.

> **NOT HUNGRY BUT NOT FULL** – she might get frustrated if she is very hungry and struggling to get to grips with the new skills required to satisfy those hunger pangs. In this case, all she will want is her usual milk. You also don't want her to be too full with no appetite for her first tastes so try and pick a time in between feeds.

> **IN A FAMILIAR, RELAXED HOME MEAL ENVIRONMENT.**

> **AT AROUND THE SAME TIME EACH DAY, TO HELP ESTABLISH A ROUTINE.**
> I would suggest introducing a new food during the day either morning or lunchtime. This also means that in the unlikely case your baby has a reaction, you can monitor and manage it in the daytime.

BEST PRACTICE

DO . . .

1. Put a small amount of food on the tip of a soft weaning spoon (if the spoon is rejected, it's OK to use the tip of a clean finger instead – although short nails are a must)

2. Place the spoon in the front of your baby's mouth so that when her lips close around it, the food is removed

3. Go really slowly, at her pace, she should be in control

DON'T . . .

1. Use your baby's upper lip or gum to scrape the food off the spoon

2. Tip the spoon to dump the food into her mouth

3. Ever use a metal spoon

4. Expect her to eat more than 1–2 teaspoons to begin with – if she is enthusiastic and wanting to take more, then see it as a bonus

good example

EATING POSITION

More often than not, for those that encounter problems with weaning, it is the position of their baby which is actually the problem – and this can easily be rectified.

The highchair must provide optimum support for their hips, knees and ankles. They should all be at 90 degree angles. Think of a capital letter 'L' if unsure what this looks like.

✓ GOOD EXAMPLE – feet supported, ankles and knees at 90 degrees and hips at 90 degrees

✗ BAD EXAMPLE – leaning back, knees not at 90 degrees and ankles swinging freely

GAGGING & CHOKING

Remember that however you are feeding your baby, she should never be left alone while eating, and she must always be supported in an upright position. It is all about going at their own pace and this will also significantly reduce the risk of choking.

It's worthwhile understanding the difference between choking and gagging as often the two can get confused and panic ensues! Gagging is your baby's own safety mechanism that prevents choking by pushing food away from the airway if it is too big to be swallowed. The gag reflex in babies is triggered towards the front of the tongue (unlike adults where this is much further back). That's why finger foods are great from 6 months because your baby learns to chew and swallow when this reflex is safely close to the front of the mouth. Choking is something very different as this is when your baby's airways become blocked. They will be unable to cry, cough, make noise or breathe and they will need immediate help.

AVOID THESE FOODS THAT COULD CAUSE CHOKING

- **Whole cherry tomatoes**
- **Whole and chopped nuts**
- **Whole grapes**
- **Fruits with stones, such as cherries**
- **Bony fish** (always check fish thoroughly for bones first)

If you are going to give grapes and cherry tomatoes, ensure they are cut up correctly. See page 46 for examples.

Babies tend to store food in their mouth for some time, so when you take them out of their highchair, just check they're not storing any spare food as a snack for later!

I encourage all new parents to become familiar with First Aid procedures for children, especially if they are concerned about choking risks when they start weaning. Refer to the Red Cross or NHS websites which have step-by-step videos or ask your GP about local First Aid courses.

---

myth buster

Babies loathe the clean-up job after a round of food exploration

It doesn't have to be so hard. Try taking baby out of their highchair and clean them up while sitting on your knee. That way, they are less likely to associate the negativity of having their face and hands wiped within their immediate feeding space (in the highchair). And, only clean them up at the end of the meal and not during. They need to be exposed to having different textures around their mouth. It's all part of the sensory experience!

FEEDING DIFFICULTIES

Did you know that around 20% of parents report feeding difficulties at some point during early childhood? These may range from eating a limited variety of food, not being interested in food, slow eating and favouring or taking a dislike to specific textures. Feeding difficulties can lead to a lot of distress for parents and for baby and can also adversely affect weight gain if they continue for a long period of time. Firstly, parents need to know that they are not alone and that feeding difficulties, whatever they may be, are extremely common. As children grow older, they challenge boundaries and start to enjoy a new-found sense of independence. Unfortunately, food is one of the first areas they realise they can control and very quickly work out that they like this feeling.

DO . . .

1. Keep mealtimes to 30 minutes and no longer

2. Avoid distraction, including TV, games and books as well as bargaining techniques

3. Offer a manageable portion as giving too much food can be overwhelming

4. Ignore bad behaviour and do not overly praise a child, if she is eating her food

5. Avoid running a restaurant service, where you offer many different meals. Most children will eventually eat, if they are hungry enough

POTENTIAL TRIGGERS FOR FEEDING PROBLEMS

Poor growth – which leads to parents wanting to feed all the time, ignoring the hunger and fullness cues of their baby. If you are worried about your baby's growth, seek the help of a dietitian or health visitor to provide you with tips on how you can increase nutrient intake without the stress.

Delaying the introduction of different textures, which may lead to gagging and choking when faced with textured foods later on.

Medical diseases that particularly affect the gastrointestinal tract (e.g. gastro-oesophageal reflux disease) and heart (congenital heart disease) can lead to feeding difficulties. These need to be managed by healthcare professionals.

Ignoring hunger and fullness cues and feeding your baby to a specific schedule irrespective of what signs she shows.

Traumatic experiences, such as an allergic reaction, can make parents reluctant to increase the variety of foods, out of fear of a future reaction.

critical nutrients

At 6 months, your baby is about to go through an amazing growth spurt. In their first year, babies triple their birth weight. To grow that much, they need a lot of nutrients – more than at any other time in their life.

Don't ever be tempted to compare your diet to your baby's, as they couldn't be more different. Be mindful that she has a tiny tummy which fills up very quickly. This means that every mouthful or spoonful she has needs to contain the maximum amount of nutrition (with minimum amount of bulk). Each meal should contain protein, carbohydrates and fat.

Here, I take the confusion out of critical nutrients, and provide a list of foods that you should be experimenting with feeding your baby.

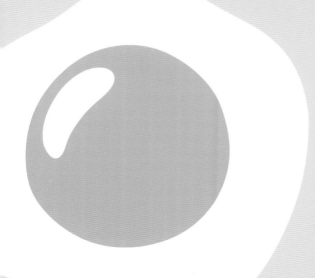

PROTEIN

Protein is an essential nutrient for growth and is most effectively used when your baby has enough energy from carbohydrates and fats, known as non-protein energy.

GOOD SOURCES OF PROTEIN FOR BABIES INCLUDE:

- **Fish** (salmon, mackerel, cod, haddock)
- **Poultry** (chicken, turkey)
- **Meat** (lamb, pork, beef)
- **Eggs** (yolks and whites)
- **Pulses like beans, lentils, chickpeas and soya** (including tofu)
- **Milk** (your baby can have full fat cow's milk in cooking from the start of weaning once over 6 months)
- **Yoghurt** (full fat)
- **Cheese**
- **Nuts** (ground or nut butters)

CARBOHYDRATES

Carbohydrates will give your baby the fuel she needs to grow and develop and will help to make the best use of the protein-based foods she is consuming. She will need carbohydrates that are easily digested by her immature digestive system.

It is really important that you choose a mixture of both white and wholegrain carbs. Options such as granary and seeded bread are fantastic sources of fibre, but too much fibre can be a little bit bulky and too filling for babies. It can even inhibit their appetite and also reduce the absorption of key nutrients, so at mealtimes try alternating between both white and wholegrain.

GOOD SOURCES OF CARBOHYDRATES FOR BABIES INCLUDE:

- **Bread** (white and wholegrain)
- **Pasta** (white and wholegrain)
- **Rice** (white and wholegrain)
- **Potatoes**
- **Sweet potatoes**
- **Cereals**
- **Grains** (bulgur wheat, quinoa)

FATS

Fats are essential to include in your baby's diet. They are easy to digest, the basis for brain growth and critical for overall growth and development. Babies should not be on a low fat diet, as plenty of good fats at this age will not make them fat or lead to heart problems in later life.

Fats are the foundation building blocks for brain tissue and contribute around 50% of your baby's energy requirements. In fact, in the first 2 years of life, your baby's brain is growing and developing at a faster rate than it will ever do again.

Foods that are high in fat such as avocados, meats, oily fish and cheese are an essential part of your baby's diet. Seeds and ground nuts can be used in baked foods such as muffins, and nut butters can be used from 6 months. You can also serve fresh fruit with full fat yoghurt and lightly fry or roast vegetables tossed with olive, sunflower or rapeseed oil. Soya and many pulses are vegetarian sources that contain fat.

ESSENTIAL FATTY ACIDS

Essential fatty acids include omega 3 and omega 6 fatty acids of which omega 3, including EPA and DHA, are the most important as most babies do not consume sufficient amounts from their diet. These are vital for the development of the retinas in the eyes as well as brain growth and development, and studies suggest children who get enough of these essential fatty acids grow up to have better cognitive skills, better social skills and fewer behaviour problems.

As it is so important in your baby's diet and is passed on through breast milk, make sure those omega 3-rich foods are on your menu too. Omega 3 is now also added to all infant formula milks for babies under 1 year of age.

Ideally you should include a serving of oily fish twice a week, but no more for baby. You can opt for salmon, mackerel, trout, herring and sardines. Unfortunately, tinned tuna does not count and if cooking fresh tuna for your baby, serve it no more than once a week due to the high mercury content.

Flax seeds, chia seeds and soya beans contain a different kind of omega 3 called ALA which the body has to convert into DHA which means it is not as beneficial as the type you get from oily fish, but it provides a little helping hand nonetheless.

GOOD SOURCES OF OMEGA 3 FOR BABIES INCLUDE:

- **Oily fish** (salmon, mackerel, sardines, anchovies)
- **Chia seeds**
- **Flax seed oil**
- **Nuts** (smooth nut butters and ground nuts, not whole or chopped nuts)

GOOD SOURCES OF GENERAL FATS FOR BABIES INCLUDE:

- **Egg yolks**
- **Avocado**
- **Coconut and coconut oil**
- **Cheese** (cow, sheep and goat's milk)
- **Yoghurt** (full fat)
- **Butter** (unsalted)
- **Unrefined oils** (olive, avocado, nut, rapeseed, soya)
- **Meat** (lamb, pork, beef – even lean meat contains fat but especially minced/ground meat with at least 15% fat)
- **Poultry** (chicken and turkey)

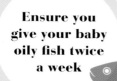

Ensure you give your baby oily fish twice a week

IRON

Iron is the micronutrient that enables the blood to carry oxygen around the body. It is required for making haemoglobin (red blood cells) and a deficiency in iron causes anaemia. It is vital for normal brain development in babies. In fact, an iron deficiency in babies between 6–12 months can impact cognitive, motor and social development skills in the future.

Full term babies are born with a reserve of iron, and until 6 months, she's been busy using the store of iron she inherited from mum. But it'll be running out by this point. While formula milk contains added iron, the absorption rate is lower than from breast milk, which has a lower content but is highly absorbable. Either way, it means that additional iron is needed and it must come from food.

The main reason a deficiency of iron may occur in babies is delaying the introduction of iron-rich foods beyond 6 months. By this age, iron-rich foods need to feature quite heavily in her diet.

If you're a meat-eating family, then be sure to introduce meat/fish from 6 months as both are full of all-important iron. She will absorb iron from meat more easily than iron from any other source, and lean beef is packed with it: the darker the flesh, the higher the iron content.

If you follow a vegetarian diet, then do not worry, there are plenty of non-meat sources of iron. However, as these are plant-based, the absorption of this form of iron is lower, so the amount required is slightly higher. Combining non-meat/fish sources of iron with vitamin C-rich foods will help the absorption of iron.

Offer a small portion of fresh fruit (for example a few strawberries) or chopped up raw veggies such as peppers or tomatoes. A squeeze of lemon at the end of cooking in a meal also works well (i.e. a lentil dhal with a squeeze of lemon). If you are cooking your vegetables then be sure to lightly cook these as vitamin C is heat sensitive and heating for a prolonged time reduces the level of this nutrient. A steamed broccoli floret is perfect here to act as her vitamin C fix.

GOOD SOURCES OF IRON FOR BABIES INCLUDE:

Haem iron (from meat/fish)

- **Meat** (beef, lamb)
- **Poultry** (the darker meat is slightly higher in iron)
- **Fish**

Non-haem iron (not from meat/fish)

- **Pulses** (lentils, kidney beans, chickpeas, soya beans)
- **Egg yolks**
- **Green leafy veggies** (spinach, broccoli, kale)
- **Fortified breakfast cereals**
- **Wholegrain foods** (pasta, bread, chia seeds)
- **Sweet potatoes** (skin on)
- **Squash and pumpkins**
- **Nut butters** (smooth peanut butter)
- **Dried fruit** (dates, apricots, raisins, cranberries)
- **Dried seeds** (sunflower, pumpkin, sesame)

VITAMIN D

Vitamin D is needed for strong teeth and bones (because it acts to absorb calcium) and it regulates the immune system. The best source is the sun, which needs exposed skin during high sunshine, although babies should not be exposed to direct sunlight without protecting their sensitive skin with clothing and sunscreen.

Only a small number of food sources apart from breast milk and fortified formula milk contain enough vitamin D for babies.

Whilst the foods listed below help with vitamin D intake, babies and children do need to take a vitamin D supplement (see page 47 for information on supplements).

SOURCES OF VITAMIN D FOR BABIES INCLUDE:

- **Oily fish** (salmon, mackerel, sardines)
- **Egg yolks**
- **Cheese**
- **Fortified foods** (margarines, milks, cereals)

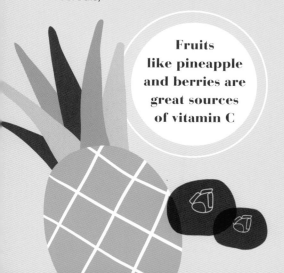

Fruits like pineapple and berries are great sources of vitamin C

VITAMIN C

The body needs vitamin C to grow, repair and heal itself. The good news is that it is the most abundant vitamin in fruit and vegetables!

GOOD SOURCES OF VITAMIN C FOR BABIES INCLUDE:

- **Mango**
- **Citrus fruits**
- **Kiwi**
- **Papaya**
- **Pineapple**
- **Berries**
- **Tomatoes**
- **Peppers**
- **Green leafy veggies** (spinach, broccoli)

Add a vitamin C-rich food to a meal to help iron absorption

VITAMIN B

The B vitamins are a group of water-soluble vitamins needed for cell energy metabolism. While B vitamins are essential, we know that generally a well-balanced diet of fresh food will be enough.

SOURCES OF VITAMIN B FOR BABIES INCLUDE:

- **Meat, poultry and fish**
- **Eggs**
- **Dairy produce**
- **All legumes**
- **Seeds and nuts**
- **Grains, in particular wholegrains** (just not too much – see the Carbohydrates section on page 38)
- **All fruit and all vegetables**

VITAMIN A

Vitamin A is a critical nutrient for healthy eye development, eyesight and a healthy immune system as well as for skin and neurological functions.

GOOD SOURCES OF VITAMIN A FOR BABIES INCLUDE:

- **Sweet potato**
- **Carrots**
- **Squash**
- **Red peppers**
- **Green leafy veggies** (spinach, broccoli, kale)
- **Apricots**
- **Mango**
- **Papaya**
- **Nectarines**
- **Guava**
- **Butter** (unsalted)
- **Eggs**
- **Oily fish**
- **Cheese**

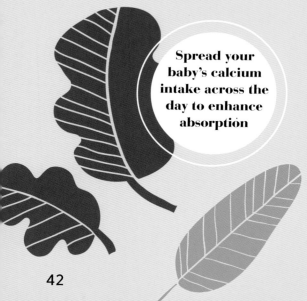

Spread your baby's calcium intake across the day to enhance absorption

CALCIUM

Calcium is essential for good bone development and important for blood to clot, nerves to send messages and muscles to work effectively. Yet calcium on its own is ineffective. Without sufficient magnesium, phosphate, vitamin K and vitamin D, the calcium consumed by your baby cannot be effectively absorbed. The greater their intake of vitamin D and these other co-factors, the less calcium they need to consume because their body will be able to absorb more.

Dairy products provide the highest sources of calcium. However, there are other non-dairy sources of calcium, but their absorption may be lower due to the lack of added co-factors like magnesium, phosphate and vitamin K.

BEST NON-MILK SOURCES OF CALCIUM FOR BABIES INCLUDE:

- **Seeds** (chia, sesame in tahini, poppy)
- **Some lentils and beans**
- **Sardines and tinned salmon** (because of the bones)
- **Almonds** (as a nut butter)
- **Some green leafy veggies** (spinach, broccoli, kale)
- **Oranges**
- **Figs**
- **Fortified foods** (including calcium enriched soya/coconut yoghurts/desserts)

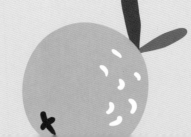

IODINE

Iodine deficiency is the most common cause worldwide for developmental delay for babies and children. Iodine intake is a particular problem among vegans and those with a milk allergy. The main source is from milk and milk products but children with milk allergies are at a clear disadvantage here as they can't up their intake from this source.

GOOD SOURCES OF IODINE FOR BABIES INCLUDE:

* **Dairy foods**
* **Fish**
* **Seaweed** (one of the highest sources of iodine)
* **Eggs**
* **Nuts** (ground or as nut butter)

ZINC

Zinc is an essential nutrient for the skin, the digestive system, supporting a heathy immune system, and in particular, growth.

The good news is that high-protein foods are the best source of zinc (see the list on page 37) and all of the iron-rich foods mentioned (see the list page 40) are also high in zinc so if your baby is getting that all-important dose of iron twice a day then she'll be getting enough zinc in her diet.

PREBIOTICS

A prebiotic is the non-digestible part of a food such as the fibre in grains, onions, garlic and artichokes that stimulate the growth and/or activity of good bacteria in a baby's gut and therefore improve their overall health.

PROBIOTICS

Probiotics are live organisms that benefit the health of babies by improving and restoring their gut bacterial flora. The importance of the bacteria in the gut has received a lot of attention over the last ten years and research shows that it could be the key to the prevention and development of many diseases, so maintaining this is important. The good news is that parents can do a lot about improving the good bacteria in the gut of their baby by introducing a variety of foods, including foods that are naturally high in probiotics, including onions, garlic, leeks, artichokes, banana, oats and barley. These may give your baby a little bit more wind the first couple of times you trial them, but don't worry as this just means that they are stimulating the growth of bacteria.

Many foods contain natural probiotics, including yoghurts, cheese and fermented cabbage (like sauerkraut). A lot of parents want to provide their baby with a probiotic supplement, but your baby has millions of different bacteria in the gut, so this can be quite a challenge and not as easy as it seems! It is therefore important to get advice from a healthcare professional on choosing the right one as the type, survival of the bacteria, and amount, is important.

NUTRIENT-RICH FOODS, AT A GLANCE

The list of foods babies can eat is long and varied, and it can be daunting knowing where to begin. So, to make things simple, I've created a quick reference guide to some of the best foods for your baby.

These provide a strong foundation for a whole host of tasty meals. You'll find most of these foods in my recipes.

Remember, first stage weaning is about your baby exploring and experimenting, so don't worry if they get spat out or thrown to the dog, persist with new tastes and textures to pave the way for an adventurous eater.

By no means is this an exhaustive list, but it works as a good reference guide.

FATS	CARBOHYDRATES	PROTEINS
Oils (olive oil, coconut oil, rapeseed oil, soya oil)	Potatoes	Chicken
	White and wholegrain pasta	Turkey
Egg yolks		Beef
Dairy (cheese, full fat yoghurt, unsalted butter)	Rice, bread and grains (bulgur wheat, oats, quinoa, corn, tapioca)	Lamb
		Pork
Oily fish (salmon, mackerel, sardines)	Fortified breakfast cereals	Salmon
		Cod
Avocados		Haddock
		Egg white
Nuts (smooth butters or ground nuts: almonds, cashews, peanuts, walnuts)		**Milk** (full fat cow's milk)
		Cheese
		Yoghurt (full fat)
		Pulses (beans, lentils, tofu)
		Nuts and seeds

TOP FOOD TIPS FOR YOUR BABY

 ## Fibre
To get your baby's fibre balance right, offer her a mixture of white and wholegrain pasta, and bread.

 ## Eggs
Eggs are full of nutrients including high quality protein and many of the vitamins and minerals essential for your baby's growth. Plus, the Food Standards Agency confirmed in October 2017 that eggs that carry the British Lion mark can safely be eaten runny, even by pregnant women and babies. *Visit egginfo.co.uk.*

 ## Fish
Ensure that oily fish, such as salmon, features on your baby's menu twice a week, but no more, due to pollutants/mercury levels, which may build up in the body and can be harmful to the brain and nervous system. Include white fish too.

 ## Yoghurt
Ensure yoghurts are unsweetened and full fat.

 ## Beans & pulses
Beans and pulses are very good sources of protein, iron and fibre (the type of fibre which is good for your baby's bowels and heart). You may need to push these through a sieve to remove hard outer husks.

 ## Fruit & vegetables
Fruit and vegetables are essential sources of vitamin C to help absorb iron whilst also providing fibre. Offer a small portion at every meal.

 ## Nutritionally complete meals
Lots of the recipes in this book are marked as 'nutritionally complete'. This means they contain a protein, carbohydrate and fruit/vegetable in one meal so the recipe provides all 'ingredients' for a perfect meal in one.

FOODS TO AVOID BEFORE 1 YEAR

Honey There is a very small chance it might contain the food poisoning bacteria botulism. This is a very serious condition but extremely rare	**Rice milk in large volumes** Contains a more concentrated form of arsenic and the long-term effects of this are unknown	**Refined sugar** As babies have a sweet tooth they will be more attracted to sweet foods and this can have health risks as she gets older
Processed foods Contain additives and E numbers	**Unpasteurised cow's milk, cheeses & yoghurts**	**Salt** A baby's kidneys can't deal with this at this age
Baby juices and herbal drinks She only needs milk and water	**Tea, coffee, chocolate, sweets, fizzy drinks**	**All forms of caffeine**

The foods below are OK for your baby, but make sure you cut these appropriately to avoid the risk of choking:

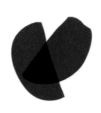

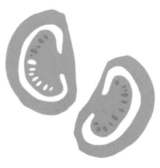

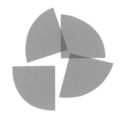

BLUEBERRIES (LARGE ONES SHOULD BE HALVED)

CHERRY TOMATOES (SHOULD BE QUARTERED)

GRAPES (SHOULD BE HALVED LENGTHWISE, THEN HALVED AGAIN)

SUPPLEMENTS

Between the ages of 6 months to 5 years the only three vitamins the Department of Health recommend supplementing are vitamins A, C, and D, unless babies and children are consuming more than 500ml of formula. For breastfed babies, it is recommended to have a vitamin D supplement from birth, irrespective of whether mum is taking a vitamin D supplement.

There are various baby vitamin products available in easy liquid form that provide these vitamins, and some contain other vitamins as well as minerals. Choose one which is free from artificial colours, flavourings, sweeteners, refined sugar and allergens.

Current recommended intake for children over 6 months. It's important to choose a supplement that has at least these 3 vitamins as ingredients

NUTRIENT	PER DAY
Vitamin A*	350 micrograms
Vitamin C*	25 milligrams
Vitamin D*	10 micrograms
Iodine	60 ug
Calcium	525 milligrams
Iron	7.8 milligrams

special diets

VEGETARIAN & VEGAN

If you are setting out to wean your baby on a vegetarian or vegan diet, then of course this is absolutely do-able, however, parents do have to be extra careful to ensure their baby's diet is well balanced and they are still getting the critical nutrients (in particular iron and B12) required for their long-term health and development.

The good news is that for the first 6 months of your baby's life, they will naturally get most of the vitamins, minerals and other nutrients they need from their regular milk. Babies weaned before 6 months start off vegetarian anyway, as vegetable and fruit purées form the basis of their diets for the first month or so. However, after these first tastes have been mastered there are some key nutritionals you need to consider.

If you want to raise your child as vegan or vegetarian, she will also need to have two portions of iron-rich protein per day (i.e. any of the pulses or nut butters) but ideally this should be combined with a food rich in vitamin C.

Take your baby to be weighed and measured at your local health centre around once a month and plot her weight and growth on the growth chart in your baby's red book (see page 70). This will give you an idea of whether she is obtaining enough nutrients from her food in order to grow and develop well.

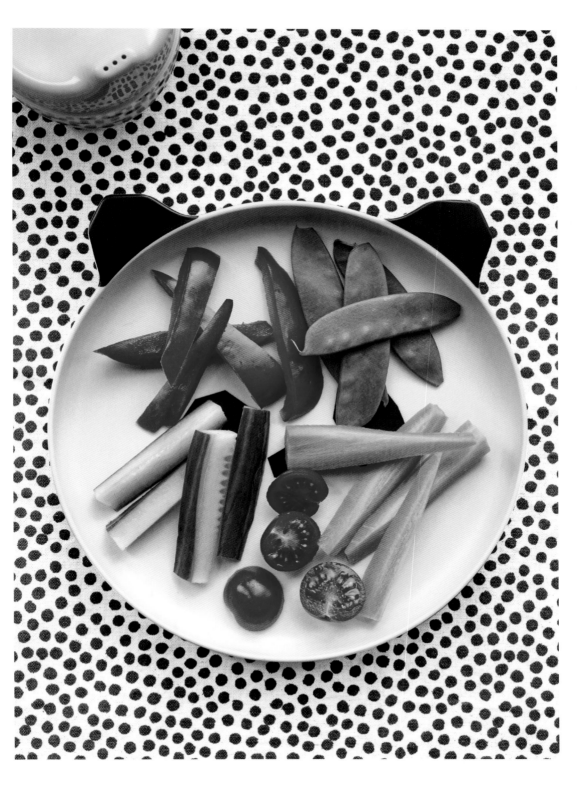

NUTRIENT	WHY IT'S IMPORTANT	VEGAN SOURCES	OTHER VEGETARIAN SOURCES
Protein	Vegetarian and vegan babies need to have a source of protein with every meal. It is needed for the growth and creation of enzymes which help to control bodily functions	Beans, lentils, chickpeas, other pulses, nuts (ground) and nut butters, seeds, soya products including tofu, tempeh and Quorn	Eggs, cheese, full fat yoghurt, milk (your baby can have full fat cow's milk in cooking from the start of weaning once over 6 months)
Omega 3	Omega 3 is in breast milk and the EU requires this to be added to infant formula milk. It is essential for optimal brain and eye development and is also thought to be linked to behaviour and intelligence	Walnuts (ground or in nut butter), tofu, rapeseed and flax seed oils *These foods contain a different form of omega 3 from that in the likes of salmon and other oily fish. Your baby will convert this into DHA and EPA, the optimal forms of omega 3. However, the conversion depends on many genetic factors and a vegan supplement may be needed. I recommend seeking advice from a dietitian*	Eggs laid by hens fed on omega 3 grains, omega 3 fortified dairy foods, such as milk and yoghurt
Iron	Iron is needed for brain development and an iron deficiency can affect behaviour, intellect and growth so it is important to ensure that vegetarian and vegan babies have two portions of iron-rich food a day. You will need to pair it with a vitamin C-rich food such as fruit or raw veggies to maximise absorption – try a few chopped blueberries (see page 46 for cutting instructions) or a lightly steamed broccoli floret alongside their iron source	Pulses (lentils, kidney beans, chickpeas, soya beans), nuts (ground) and nut butters, seeds, green leafy vegetables, squash and pumpkin, soya products including tofu, unsalted seitan, fortified breakfast cereals, dried fruit, wholegrains, tahini and blackcurrants	Egg yolks

NUTRIENT	WHY IT'S IMPORTANT	VEGAN SOURCES	OTHER VEGETARIAN SOURCES
Iodine	Needed for thyroid function which makes hormones, regulates metabolism, heart rate, body temperature and how she regulates energy from food. It is also involved in brain development. Iodine deficiency can be a real problem in both vegan adults and children	Most vegan babies will obtain enough from **breast** or **formula milk**. If they are taking less than 500ml per day, a supplement may be required – seek advice from a dietitian before choosing one	**Dairy foods**. It is rare for vegetarian babies to not get enough iodine
Selenium	An antioxidant that can help protect the body from damage caused by free radicals and also helps to control the speed of reactions in the body. Selenium is also needed for thyroid health	Most vegan babies get enough from **breast milk** or **formula** but may need a supplement if their intake is less than 500ml per day **Brazil nuts** (ground), **cashew nuts, lentils, brown rice, sunflower seeds, baked beans, mushrooms, oats, spinach, bananas**	**Eggs, milk** and **milk products**
Zinc	Needed for her immune system, growth and metabolism and creating DNA. It is involved in wound healing and the development of taste and energy regulation. Zinc is less well absorbed from plant sources so vegan babies must have zinc-containing foods every day	**Wholegrain carbohydrate foods** – **bread, pasta, rice** and other **grains** (see page 38, Carbohydrates section, for an important note on fibre) **nuts** and **seeds, leafy and root vegetables, fermented soya products** such as **miso** or **unsalted tempeh, beans**	**Eggs, dairy**

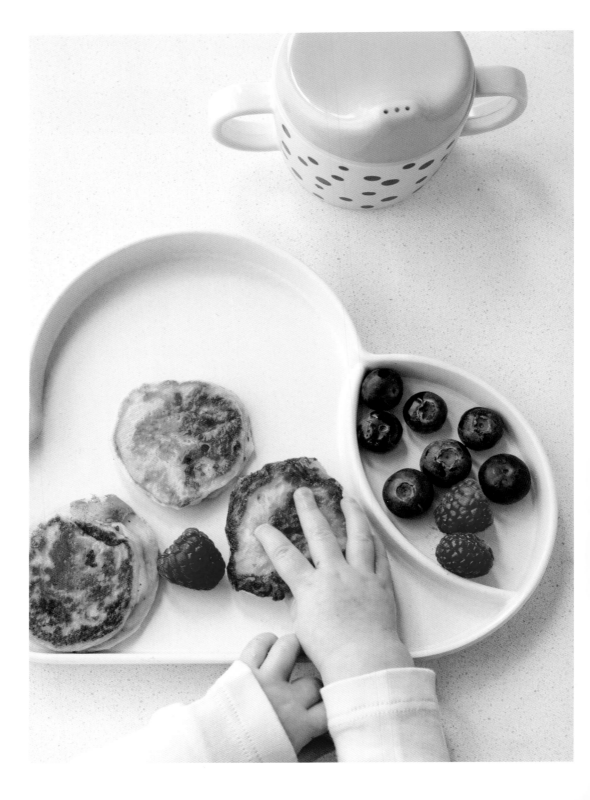

NUTRIENT	WHY IT'S IMPORTANT	VEGAN SOURCES	OTHER VEGETARIAN SOURCES
Vitamin B12	Essential for the central nervous system and the formulation of red blood cells. A deficiency can result in a type of anaemia. Most vegan babies will need a supplement but seek advice from a dietitian first. If vegan mums are taking a vitamin B12 supplement, it can pass through into the breast milk in adequate amounts. Formula is fortified with it	**Fortified foods** e.g. some **breakfast cereals** and **plant milks**, also **yeast extract** such as **Marmite** (although this is very salty and unsuitable for babies)	Eggs, dairy
Calcium	Essential for healthy bone development, nerve and muscle function. It is the combination of calcium, magnesium, vitamin K2, D and phosphate (which you get in milk products) that leads to an optimal bone density. Vitamin D is needed in order for calcium to be absorbed	**Fortified foods** e.g. **plant milks, tofu, green vegetables, almond butter, tahini, lentils, beans, oranges, figs** and **seeds** If you live in a hard water area calcium may be in your **tap water** too	Eggs, dairy
Vitamin D	Needed so calcium can be absorbed. Sunshine is the key for all of us, babies and adults alike! It forms vitamin D in our skin but in the UK we don't receive enough sunlight. Babies should not be exposed to direct sunlight without protecting their sensitive skin with clothing and sunscreen. All babies need a vitamin D supplement of 10 micrograms/day	**Fortified foods** e.g. some **margarines, orange juice** and **breakfast cereals**	Eggs, dairy

allergies

Childhood food allergies are on the increase, so it's natural that some parents might be nervous about introducing foods that have the potential to cause problems. But it's good to note that the actual incidence of food allergy in babies is very low – about 3–6%. And the good news is that babies and children tend to grow out of allergies such as cow's milk or an egg allergy by the age of 3–5 years.

Food allergies are more common amongst children from families where other members suffer from an allergy, but this is because this increases the risk of eczema, and babies who suffer from eczema are at a higher risk of having food allergies. The more severe the eczema and the earlier in life that it began, the more likely there is to be a food allergy. However, specific food allergies are not inherited.

There are two types of allergic reaction – immediate onset (usually within 2 hours) and delayed onset (2 hours–2 days). This is why parents often like to introduce potential allergen foods early in the day so they can observe their baby throughout the day for any signs.

SIGNS OF IMMEDIATE ONSET ALLERGIC REACTION	SIGNS OF DELAYED ONSET ALLERGIC REACTION
<ul><li>Acute vomiting</li><li>Red rash</li><li>Hives</li><li>Eczema</li><li>Swelling of mouth or face</li><li>Wheezing</li><li>**Anaphylaxis** – requires urgent medical attention. Symptoms include breathing difficulties, sudden pallor, sudden drowsiness, swelling of the throat and around the face and collapse</li></ul>	<ul><li>Diarrhoea</li><li>Constipation</li><li>Blood in the stools</li><li>Gastro-oesophageal reflux disease (chronic vomiting with pain)</li><li>**Colic type symptoms,** in association with other allergic symptoms</li><li>Eczema</li><li>**Poor weight gain** in association with other symptoms above</li></ul>

WEANING WITH ALLERGIES

For babies who don't have parents or siblings with allergies, or who don't have early-onset eczema, start introducing solids the normal way. You don't need to offer the allergenic foods differently to other foods. However, if you think your baby is at risk of food allergy, it may be sensible to discuss this with your GP before you start weaning.

The most common causes of the immediate type of food allergy are cow's milk, egg, soy, wheat, sesame, peanuts, fish, shellfish and tree nuts. With delayed allergies, milk and soya are the most common causes. It is worth being aware of these common top allergenic foods when you are weaning your baby and introducing them to new foods.

the most common allergens Food Standards Agency

1. Cow's milk

2. Hen's eggs

3. Peanuts (a legume rather than a nut)

4. Tree nuts (almonds, cashews, hazelnuts etc)

5. Fish

6. Shellfish (prawns, crab etc)

7. Sesame

8. Soya

9. Wheat

10. Celery

11. Molluscs (mussels, oysters etc)

12. Sulphur dioxide (preservative used in dried fruits such as raisins, dried apricots etc)

13. Mustard

14. Lupin (a flower and often found in flour)

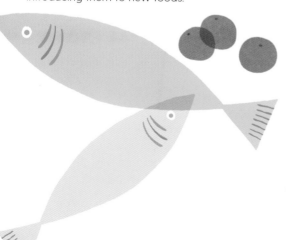

INTRODUCING ALLERGENS

New advice is not to withhold foods like eggs or peanuts from 6 months as giving these foods can help to desensitise babies. In fact, studies have shown that an early introduction of the common allergenic foods can reduce the development of these allergies.

Current advice is to ideally exclusively breastfeed for 6 months and then, between 6–12 months, to introduce appropriate solid foods (including egg and peanut) one by one into her weaning diet alongside ongoing breastfeeding. Once introduced, these foods can make up part of her normal diet. However, if there is a high risk of food allergy, such as significant eczema, it is advisable to discuss the introduction of solid foods with your doctor.

It is really important not to delay offering these foods beyond 12 months of age as research suggests this may increase the likelihood of developing an allergy in the future (there is a critical window in being able to accept potential allergenic foods from around 6 months to 12 months).

Anaphylaxis

If your baby has symptoms of an allergic reaction that affects her breathing and/or causes lethargy and/or reduced consciousness, call an ambulance immediately or go to your local A&E department. This may be an anaphylactic reaction, which can cause a drop in blood pressure and/or tightening or swelling in the airway.

myth buster

Avoid offering foods a parent is allergic/intolerant to

You should not be avoiding a food you or a family member is allergic or intolerant to. New research in fact supports an early introduction of allergens. However, it is worth having a discussion with an allergist or a dietitian on how to do this safely if another family member has an allergy. In the case of food intolerances (which are rare in early childhood), where life-threatening reactions do not occur, foods should be introduced as part of a weaning diet and your baby monitored to assess tolerance.

Cow's milk allergy

Cow's milk protein allergy is one of the most common childhood food allergies, estimated to affect around 1.3% of babies aged under one. The good news is that most children grow out of it by the age of five. It typically develops when cows' milk is first introduced to your baby's diet either in formula or when you start to wean your baby. It can also affect babies who are exclusively breastfeeding, because of cow's milk protein from the mother's diet passing on to the baby through breast milk, but this is not that common.

Cow's milk protein allergy can cause symptoms such as eczema, colic, reflux, diarrhoea or, if it is the immediate type of reaction, then hives or rarely, anaphylaxis (see page 54 for a list of symptoms). Many typical features of a milk allergy are actually common symptoms in a completely healthy baby so it is important not to overinterpret these. Typically, milk allergy is more likely if the symptoms are severe, persistent, multiple and resistant to treatment and it is at this point that it may be worth discussing the possibility with your doctor.

➤ **Milk substitute hypoallergenic formula** For the first year, ideally breast milk is given to infants but when this isn't possible, formula milk is given as cow's milk does not provide adequate iron and other nutrients until 1 year. However, infant formula is made from cow's milk so if your baby has a cow's milk allergy this means they will need a special hypoallergenic formula that is extensively hydrolysed or amino-acid based (available on prescription).

In the first year, babies who are not breastfed will need ideally 600ml of hypoallergenic formula a day to meet their nutritional requirements.

➤ **Plant-based milks** such as oat, almond, cashew, flax, hemp, rice and coconut are not suitable milk alternatives for children under 2 as they are very low in energy, protein, fats, vitamin D and iodine. Using a small amount in cooking is fine but otherwise they are best avoided. If these are used after 1 year of age as your baby's main drink, dietary adequacy ideally needs to be assessed by a dietitian.

Soya milk should not be used under 6 months of age as a milk formula in children with a cow's milk allergy, and after this age, it should be noted that up to 50% of children with a delayed cow's milk allergy may also react to soya. See your GP with any concerns or ask for a referral to a paediatric dietitian for more advice.

You will also need to avoid rice milk until 4½ years of age. Although it's unlikely that you'll be offering your baby rice milk in large quantities, you need to be careful of this dairy-free alternative as it contains a high level of arsenic which is found in the soil and can accumulate in rice at a higher level than in other grains. Don't worry about other rice products such as rice cakes and rice as these are perfectly safe for your baby to have before 12 months, it's just the rice milk you need to avoid as this is a more concentrated form and we don't yet know the long-term effects.

NOTE: *Partially hydrolysed formulas (available without prescription), where proteins are broken down to make them less allergenic, are not suitable for babies with Cow's Milk Protein Allergy (CMPA).*

Always consult your GP or a registered dietitian with experience in children's nutrition to get a proper diagnosis and advice about ongoing cow's milk avoidance.

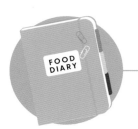

FOOD
DIARY

KEEPING A FOOD DIARY

If there is a history of allergy in the family, then it might be a good idea to keep a record of the most common allergens milk, egg, soya, wheat, fish, shellfish, peanut and tree nuts, sesame) when these are introduced and any reactions your baby has. If you have allergies in the family or if your baby has eczema, it is advisable to wait 48 hours between the introduction of the potentially allergenic foods to see if there is a reaction. So, try dairy produce, for example, and then wait for two days before introducing eggs. It is a good idea to introduce new foods at breakfast or lunchtime, so you can monitor your baby's reaction during the day.

Milk ladder

A milk ladder (where cow's milk and dairy products are gradually introduced into the diet) is based on the principle that heating and fermentation makes the milk protein less allergenic and that you can move a baby that is becoming tolerant to cow's milk 'up the ladder' from baked and highly fermented products to pasteurised milk, which is the most allergenic.

A milk ladder is ONLY suitable for children with a delayed cow's milk allergy (also called a non-IgE mediated allergy) and should not be used in a baby with an immediate (also called IgE mediated) cow's milk allergy. It's also important to discuss with your dietitian or doctor when the right time would be to introduce the milk ladder as this varies from baby to baby.

Egg allergy

Being allergic to eggs is much more common in young children than in adults, but most children will outgrow it. However, children with an egg allergy are also at a high risk of developing a peanut allergy, so they should be seen by a doctor experienced in childhood allergies.

An egg allergy can be to all forms of egg, however, research has found that 70–80% of children with an egg allergy can eat cakes and biscuits that contain baked egg, but in those who do react, the reactions can be severe.

A child with an egg allergy should be tested by an experienced doctor before eating any foods containing baked egg. This may need to be done under direct medical supervision.

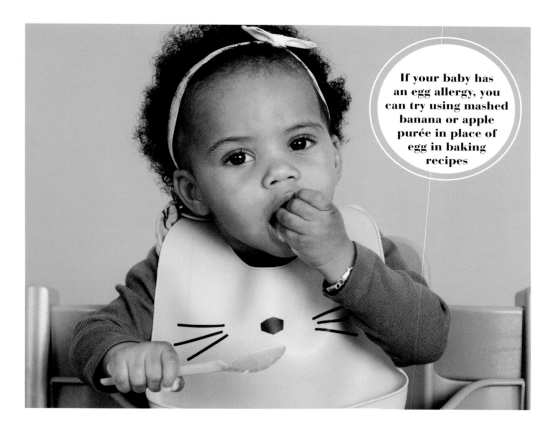

If your baby has an egg allergy, you can try using mashed banana or apple purée in place of egg in baking recipes

did you know?

Replacements in baking (equivalent of 1 egg)
- 65g apple purée
- 1 small mashed banana (roughly 65g)
- 1 tbsp vinegar and 1 tsp baking powder
- 2 tbsp arrowroot and 1 tsp baking soda

Egg replacements for binding recipes
- 60g yoghurt or buttermilk (if no milk allergy)
- Cornflour with sparkling water
- Chia seeds or flax seeds mixed with water: 1 tbsp seeds to 3 tbsp water
- Aquafaba (tinned chickpea liquid): 3 tbsp for 1 whole egg or egg white – you can use this to make pancakes and meringues

59

Nut allergy

About one in 50 children in the UK has a nut allergy. A child has a higher risk of developing a peanut allergy if she already has an allergic condition, such as eczema or a diagnosed food allergy such as to egg. Peanuts, peanut products, and tree nuts can induce a severe allergic reaction, so if you are worried have a discussion with your GP or dietitian rather than just avoiding them.

The advice on giving nuts has changed: for babies, peanut butter and finely ground nuts can be introduced from 6 months. Those with a high risk of allergy, for example due to significant eczema, may wish to discuss this with your doctor.

The advice used to be that a child allergic to peanuts should avoid all nuts completely. However, there is concern that some children who do this may develop an allergy to nuts they were not allergic to because they avoided eating them at a critical time. You should get tailored advice around this from the doctor/dietitian who diagnoses the allergy.

Tree nuts, such as cashews, pecans, walnuts, pistachio, and almonds, are not related to peanuts but can also cause reactions. You may be advised not to give other nuts to your child if your child is allergic to peanuts. Whole nuts should be avoided until five years of age due to the risk of choking.

Wheat allergy & coeliac disease

A wheat allergy is uncommon and when found this is usually in children who have eczema and/or multiple food allergies. It is usually outgrown in childhood.

Coeliac disease, which is hereditary, is different from an allergy to wheat. It is an autoimmune condition triggered by a protein called gluten in certain grains (wheat, oat, rye and barley). Symptoms include chronic diarrhoea, tiredness, tummy ache, iron deficiency, faltering growth, and offensive-smelling poo. It is diagnosed by a blood test and endoscopy, but your child needs to be having wheat in her diet when tested so always see the doctor before you cut it out. Unfortunately, gluten can be hidden in food such as soups, sauces, fish fingers, chicken nuggets, and salad dressings.

It's important not to cut wheat or gluten out of your child's diet unnecessarily as she may then be at risk of developing deficiencies in energy, B vitamins, and fibre.

When looking for wheat alternatives, it is vitally important to check the labelling on packaging. Gluten-free doesn't mean wheat free. Sometimes a product may contain the rest of the wheat grain with just the gluten removed. People with coeliac disease can only eat foods labelled as 'gluten-free' as even traces of gluten can cause problems. If your child has coeliac disease, check food labels carefully or use the Coeliac UK food scanner app. Don't just assume the food is safe as many naturally gluten-free foods can be cross-contaminated.

For more information about coeliac disease, refer to the Coeliac UK website, coeliac.org.uk.

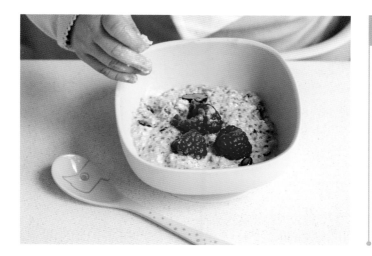

Gluten-free oats are now allowed in gluten-free diets

It is recognised that oat gluten is different from wheat, rye, and barley gluten. However, people with coeliac disease should buy gluten-free oats to avoid those that may have been contaminated by gluten during processing.

Gluten-free substitutes

You can substitute plain wheat-containing flour for wheat-free and gluten-free flours. However, it is generally best to substitute where there is a low ratio of flour to other ingredients as then you are less reliant on gluten to hold the mixture together. Always grease and line cake tins well – gluten-free baked products tend to be more fragile.

- When you are baking, use xanthan gum with gluten-free flour to enhance the texture so that the finished product is less crumbly.

- Crushed cornflakes or Rice Krispies make a good coating for home-made fish fingers or chicken nuggets, but not all are gluten-free so do check carefully.

- Gluten-free panko (Japanese) breadcrumbs.

- There are many gluten-free and wheat-free breads, crackers, pasta and pizza bases available in supermarkets.

- Rice noodles are a good substitute for pasta.

- Rice flour, polenta, buckwheat, cornflour, tapioca, arrowroot and potato flour are all naturally gluten-free so are suitable for coeliacs.

- Quinoa, millet, tapioca, amaranth and rice are good alternatives to grains.

- Cornflour and soya flour.

- Ground almonds work well in biscuits, cakes, breads and doughs.

reflux, constipation & diarrhoea

Gastrointestinal problems are actually quite common, particularly in early infancy, when breast or bottle feeding and then also with the introduction of foods, so don't be alarmed. Much of this is simply her getting used to digesting and absorbing these new nutrients.

Some of the carbohydrates in food draw water into the bowel which can cause a slightly runnier stool – not diarrhoea. Carbohydrates can also ferment in her tummy causing wind and pain. Don't panic as this is usually temporary until your baby's digestive system adapts to these new foods.

When your baby is unwell

If you think your baby is unwell, trust your instinct and seek professional help. You can get early childhood functional gastrointestinal disorders, which include reflux, constipation, colic and diarrhoea that are not explained by the gastrointestinal maturation of a baby. Doctors now have specific criteria for diagnosing these, called the Rome IV criteria, which helps them to distinguish between worrying and not-worrying symptoms. These criteria also provide very clear guidance on how to distinguish between constipation in a toilet-trained baby versus a baby in nappies. It is therefore worth seeking help quickly.

If she seems to be off her food then you can offer her more formula or breastfeeds. Additional water in between bottle feeds may also be useful. If she doesn't seem to want milk feeds then book in an appointment to see your GP or healthcare professional as you need be careful that your baby doesn't get dehydrated.

Diarrhoea

This isn't when her stool is slightly looser as mentioned above (her learning to digest different carbohydrates). Instead, diarrhoea is when her stool appears very watery and you have a frequency of 4 or more stools per day and you will certainly notice the smell! Diarrhoea is a sign of a possible viral or bacterial infection, often called gastroenteritis.

If this is the case then you will need to book in an appointment with your GP as you need to avoid dehydration. Babies are small and take small quantities of food and drink relative to their size so they can dehydrate quickly. While you are waiting for your appointment, it is important to maintain hydration so offer water in between her usual feeds (you may also need rehydration solution if the diarrhoea is very bad), or more frequent breastfeeds. Keep food simple – avoid too much fruit (no fruit juice) and try starchy foods like toast (not wholegrain) and protein, which will be kind on her tummy.

Constipation

Developing a harder stool that is less frequent can be common when you first start offering her solid food, so it is important to keep an eye on the amount of fluid she is drinking as often this can quite easily be rectified by upping her fluid intake. Remember that foods such as yoghurt/vegetable and fruit purées will help to contribute to her overall fluid intake. Fibre-rich vegetables, pulses and wholegrain foods also contain fibre – really useful in constipation as it helps to bulk out the stool and move it along the digestive system. However, too many wholegrain products may impact on her absorption of vitamins and minerals.

You can also give the 'cycling legs' method a go (when you gently begin to move your baby's legs as if she is riding a bicycle) along with a gentle tummy massage which can help to ease the symptoms.

It is important to be able to distinguish between harder stools and constipation. Constipation is defined as producing hard stools with discomfort and pain twice or less per week. If your baby does this, it is important to seek medical advice.

Reflux

You will be relieved to hear that reflux is also very common too. Your little one will bring up a small amount of milk after feeds and this is completely normal as it can take a few months for the bottom of your baby's food pipe (the lower oesophageal sphincter) to fully form.

However, if larger amounts of milk are being brought up, in particular if they are forceful and painful leading to crying with back-arching and/or positioning the head and body in an unnatural way to avoid pain, this is called gastro-oesophageal reflux disease and this will need input from your health visitor or GP, or ask for a referral to a registered dietitian.

SOME KEY SIGNS OF REFLUX ARE:

- Arching back
- Refusing feeds
- Crying
- Frequent vomiting
- Discomfort
- Poor weight gain

preparing your baby's meals

Making your own purées and baby food from scratch is not only super-satisfying but it will save you money. Most importantly, you'll know exactly what your baby is munching on at mealtimes. You'll also have full control over flavour and texture which means you can explore a world of foods to help give your baby the healthiest start.

However, it often feels like there is so much to consider when starting out – questions around sterilising, freezing and reheating and what kitchen equipment you actually need regularly crop up, so here is my step-by-step stress-free guide to preparing your own baby food!

EQUIPMENT

Most of the equipment you require will already be in your kitchen (for example, mashers, graters and sieves), but the following 10 pieces may not be, and I consider them to be key!

➤ **Electric hand blender**
This is easy to clean and ideal for making small quantities of baby purée.

➤ **Food processor**
This is good for puréeing larger quantities when making batches for freezing.

➤ **Steamer**
Steaming food is one of the best ways to preserve nutrients. It is worth buying a multi-tiered steamer but a basket over a saucepan with a well-fitting lid is a cheaper alternative.

➤ **Ice-cube trays with lids or small lidded weaning pots and re-useable pouches**
Ideal for freezing small portions or filling with home-made baby purées.

➤ **Potato ricer**
Using a standard potato masher won't give you a uniform enough texture and any surprise lumps won't be welcomed!

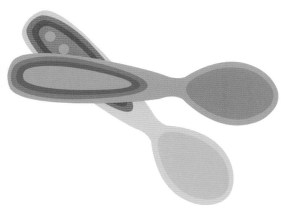

➤ Weaning spoons

Find one that features an easy grip handle and with a soft tip that is gentle on teeth and gums. You will need several spoons.

➤ Bibs with sleeves

Because let's face it, weaning is messy! Look for one with a springy, flip-out pocket to catch any food which will undoubtedly miss the mouth! Neoprene baby bibs are great as they are naturally waterproof, stretchy and soft, tough and durable.

➤ Splash mat or machine washable blanket

Particularly good if you are baby-led weaning! Even an old shower curtain placed under her highchair will do.

➤ Plastic cup – open or with lid and spout

Introduce a cup for drinks to go alongside her meals and from 6 months milk should also be offered in a cup. Avoid non-spill valved cups as these encourage your baby to use their mouth muscles in an unnatural way which is suspected to lead to speech delay. Opt for one with side grip handles to make it easier for your baby to use herself.

HOW TO COOK

Steaming, microwaving and baking are the best methods to preserve nutrients in fruit and vegetables.

➤ Steaming

This is the best way to preserve the fresh taste and vitamins. Cook your fruit and vegetables for the shortest time possible, using the least amount of water to retain nutrients. Vitamins B and C are water soluble and can easily be destroyed by over-cooking, especially when foods are boiled in water. Broccoli loses over 60% of its antioxidants when boiled, but less than 7% when streamed.

➤ Microwaving

Place the vegetables or fruit in a suitable dish. Add a little water, cover, leaving an air vent and cook on full power until tender (stirring halfway through). Purée to the desired consistency but always be sure to allow it to stand after heating, check that it isn't too hot to serve to your baby and stir well to avoid hot spots.

➤ Baking

If you're cooking a family meal in the oven, bake a sweet potato or butternut squash for your baby. Just bake until tender and then cut in half, scoop out the flesh and mash with milk to thin down to the desired consistency. Don't thin with water as it will dilute the nutrient content.

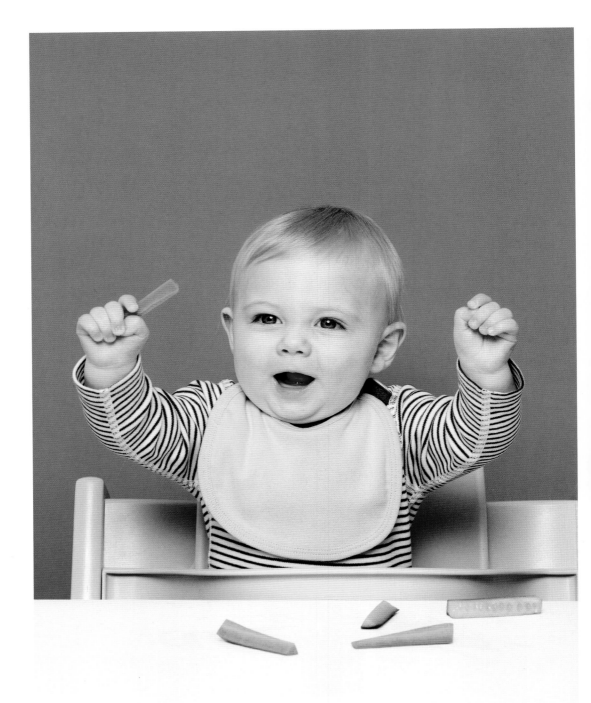

CHOOSING YOUR HIGHCHAIR

Introducing solid food is a big milestone, and your baby's highchair has a part to play in ensuring a comfy weaning ride. Here are some tips on what to look for.

No distractions

Eating is a difficult skill to learn so her focus must be 100% on the task in hand. A good highchair will ensure she isn't distracted by trying to keep herself supported instead.

Wide tray with lip

Weaning is all about play and exploration, particularly at the beginning, so choose a highchair that has a wide tray and a lip or ridge around the edge. They'll be spending lots of time smearing and smothering the tray with food, so if you have a big surface with a lip, there's less chance of them decorating the floor with their food cast-offs.

Table talk

You want to ensure that you are getting little one involved in family mealtimes, so having a highchair that can be adjusted so that your baby can be pulled right up to the table is a real positive. Look for a highchair where the tray can be removed so that your baby can use the table top directly.

Easy to clean

It's going to be a good few months before your baby's mastered those all-important coordination skills. And let's face it, food will be a whole new ball game for your baby at the beginning – especially if foods are placed directly in front of them to explore, so be prepared for a daily clean-up. Pick a highchair that is wipe clean. Ideally, look for removable straps to make cleaning them easier.

Grow together

Babies grow faster in their first year than at any other stage of life, so you'll want a highchair that grows with them. Go for a highchair that grows with your baby as they develop. After all, the last thing you want to do is invest in multiple highchairs.

Quick fold

Let's face it; babies come with a lot of stuff! But there's no need to have your highchair on show 24-7. Find one that can be easily folded up between use, and quickly set up for when you have a hungry baby wanting to eat.

FREEZING AND REHEATING

Your baby's immune system has not yet completely developed and so she will be a little more susceptible to food poisoning bacteria than adults and children. This just means you need to be slightly more aware when preparing your baby's food. Here are some of my top do's and don'ts.

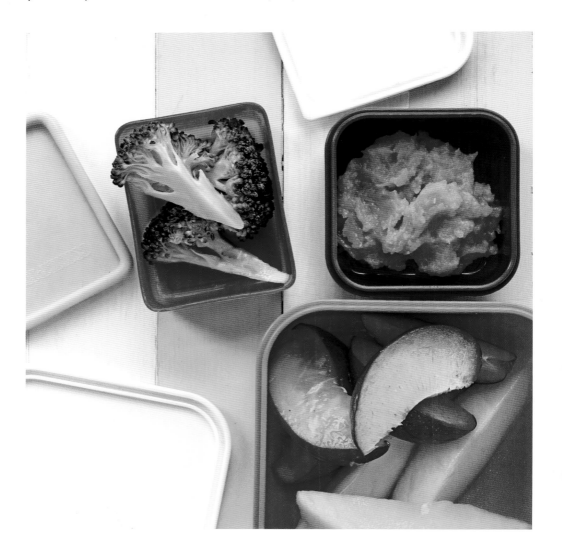

DO . . .

1. Allow your freshly made batch of purée to cool completely and freeze on the day it is cooked

2. Freeze in ice cube trays and fill these trays right up to the top. Buy trays with lids or double wrap in clingfilm to prevent contamination

3. As soon as the cubes of food are frozen, pop them out into freezer bags to reuse your trays and prevent freezer burn

4. Label and date your freezer bags. The food won't 'go off' but may degrade if left longer than 8 weeks

5. Be mindful that puréed foods don't last as long as whole foods so if your baby isn't going to eat it straight away then freeze it or use within 48 hours provided it has been in the fridge for all of this time

6. Defrost thoroughly whether by allowing to come to room temperature or on the hob or in the microwave

7. When reheating, always heat food until piping hot – this is to ensure the eradication of any food poisoning bacteria that might have grown

8. Allow hot food to cool before serving to baby

9. Use defrosted food for up to 24 hours of being out of the freezer – store defrosted food in the fridge

10. Use the top rack of the dishwasher to clean your baby's spoons and bowls (this is the hottest part) or wash by hand in hot water from the tap that is too hot without rubber gloves on

DON'T . . .

1. Refreeze defrosted food

2. Freeze leftovers from your baby's bowl or where your baby's spoon has made contact, as bacteria from her mouth will have been transferred

3. Feel the need to sterilise spoons, food containers or other feeding equipment as at this stage baby is picking up lots of things and putting these in her mouth, but everything should still be scrupulously clean

baby's red book

Your baby doesn't come with an instruction manual (unfortunately), so the Red Book (officially called the Personal Child Health Record) is the closest you'll get – aside from this book of course, which has you covered for baby's first year of food exploration!

This will be given to you by your hospital or health visitor within a week of your baby being born. You'll need it until your teeny newborn is 4 years old, so find a safe place to keep it as you'll need to dig it out for every appointment with your GP, clinic or health visitor. And if you ever need to go to A&E with your baby (hopefully not), they will need this to get an overview of baby's history.

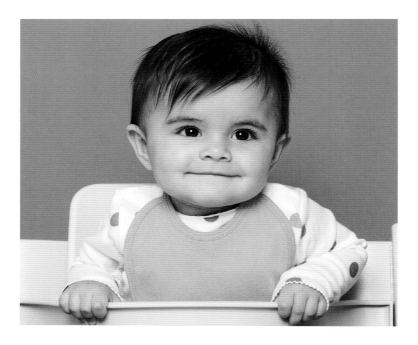

WHAT'S INSIDE YOUR RED BOOK?

Baby details and local information
This lists all the obvious things – your baby's name, NHS number and date of birth plus family contacts and details of your birth experience. There are also useful local contacts.

Immunisations
Here you'll find a list of all the vaccinations your baby will be having and when – right the way through to 4 years old. Every time they have a jab the nurse will record it in the Red Book. This helps you keep track of what they've had and when so you can keep up to date.

Screening and routine reviews
They'll be having hearing and sight checks plus regular routine health reviews, and all the results will be recorded here.

Growth charts
Don't worry, your health visitor will help you track your baby's progress on the growth charts as they are a little scary at first!

Every time your baby is weighed and measured, this will get marked on their growth chart. It's a great way to see how your baby is progressing.

Centiles explained
The growth chart is divided into centiles, which are basically just a way of comparing your baby's growth pattern to the growth pattern of babies that were exclusively breastfed and had foods introduced around 6 months of age. So if your baby is on the 25th centile for weight and the 50th for height, it means that if you lined up 100 babies from lightest to heaviest, yours would be number 25 (24 would be lighter and 75 would be heavier). For height, your baby would be number 50 – bang on average – with 49 shorter and 50 taller. All children are different and it really doesn't matter which centile your child is on – all the health professionals are looking for is that they stay roughly around the same centile for weight and length as they grow up.

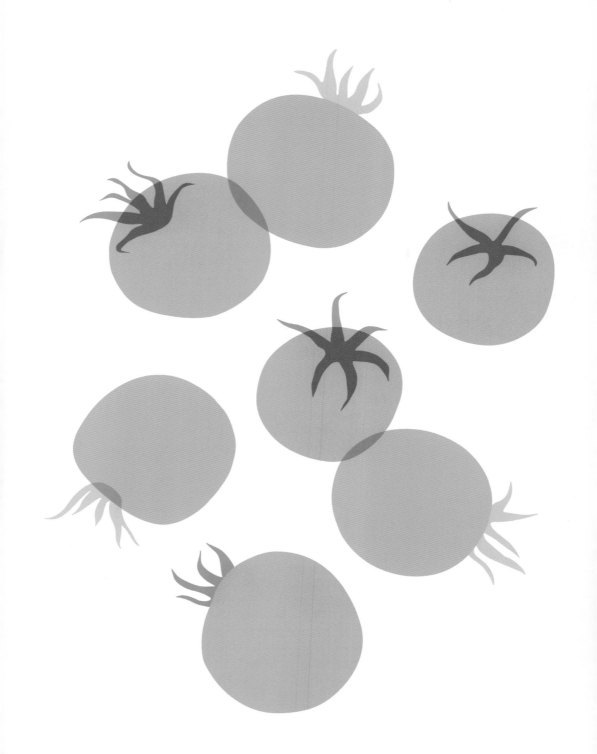

chapter 2
first tastes

first taste purées & finger foods

Whether you have opted to go down the spoon-led or baby-led route (see page 20), or maybe even a mixture of the two, your baby's actual 'first tastes' will be the same. From around 6 months your baby will start off exploring vegetables and fruits, the only difference being that you might purée these or offer as soft finger foods. So, to make it simple, I want to start by including some straightforward first taste food preparation guides, taking the same ingredient but showing how to serve as a finger food and how to purée.

It's important to note that those very first days are about introducing new tastes. And whether you're puréeing, offering finger foods, or doing a bit of both, these will be entirely new textures for your baby so they will only be having a very small amount at first – but a taste is all they need and just you wait... these initial responses are all part of the fun!

myth buster

Stick to the foods your baby likes

It's true that babies like familiar foods, so they may not like something the first time you offer it. But food habits are formed early, so if you keep offering a range of nutritious, wholesome foods, there's more chance they'll eat healthily when they're older.

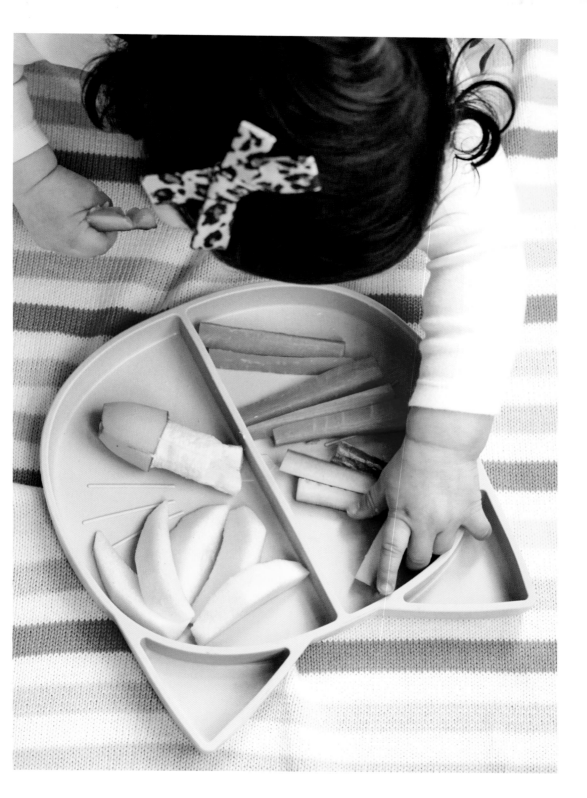

vegetables

BROCCOLI & CAULIFLOWER

Finger food
Wash the broccoli or cauliflower and cut into small florets. Steam for about 8 minutes until tender.

Purée
Steamed broccoli or cauliflower are good mixed with root vegetables like sweet potato, carrot or butternut squash. Purée with an electric stick blender or in a food processor, adding a little water from the bottom of the steamer or some of your baby's usual milk, until you reach the desired consistency.

nutritional benefits
- *Broccoli provides vitamin C, vitamin A, some B vitamins and calcium*
- *Cauliflower provides vitamin C, folic acid and some B vitamins*
- *Both are good sources of prebiotic foods*

GREEN BEANS & MANGETOUT

Finger food
Wash, top and tail the beans or mangetout. Steam for about 8 minutes until tender.

Purée
Mix steamed green beans or mangetout with root vegetables like sweet potato, carrot or butternut squash. Purée with an electric stick blender or in a food processor, adding a little water from the bottom of the steamer or some of your baby's usual milk, until you reach the desired consistency.

nutritional benefits
- *Provides vitamin C*

COURGETTE

Finger food
Wash the courgette, top and tail and cut into sticks approximately 6–7cm long and 1cm wide. Steam until tender (approximately 7 minutes).

Purée
Mix steamed courgette with root vegetables like sweet potato, carrot or butternut squash. Purée with an electric stick blender or in a food processor, adding a little water from the bottom of the steamer or some of your baby's usual milk, until you reach the desired consistency.

nutritional benefits
Provides vitamin C and some B vitamins

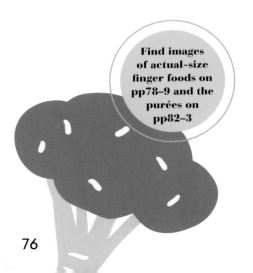

Find images of actual-size finger foods on pp78–9 and the purées on pp82–3

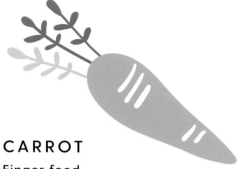

CARROT

Finger food

Peel a medium carrot and cut into sticks approximately 6–7cm long and 1cm wide. Steam for about 8 minutes or until tender. Alternatively steam baby carrots.

Purée

Dice peeled carrots and steam for 15-20 minutes or until tender. Purée with an electric stick blender or in a food processor, adding a little water from the bottom of the steamer or some of your baby's usual milk, until you reach the desired consistency.

nutritional benefits
- *Provides vitamin A*

BUTTERNUT SQUASH & PUMPKIN

Finger food
Bake
Roasting root vegetables in the oven brings out their natural sweetness. Both butternut squash and pumpkin make good weaning foods, they are unlikely to cause an allergy and are easily digested. Pop sticks or cubes of them in the oven when you are making a meal for the family.

Preheat the oven to 200°C (fan 180°C/gas mark 6). Lay a piece of foil on a baking tray, brush with sunflower, rapeseed or light olive oil. Cut the butternut squash or pumpkin in half, scoop out the seeds and fibrous strings and discard. Peel and cut into sticks approximately 6–7cm long and 1cm wide or cut into 1.5cm cubes. Arrange the veggie sticks or cubes on the lined tray and coat with oil. Bake for 15–20 minutes.

Steam
Prepare cubes or sticks of squash or pumpkin as above. Place in a steamer and steam for 12–15 minutes or until tender.

Purée
Steam
Purée steamed cubes with an electric stick blender or in a food processor, adding a little water from the bottom of the steamer or some of your baby's usual milk, until you reach the desired consistency.

Roast
Preheat the oven to 200°C (fan 180°C/gas mark 6). Line a baking tray with baking parchment. Halve the squash and scoop out the seeds and fibrous strings from both halves. Brush the cut sides with sunflower, rapeseed or light olive oil. Place cut side down on the lined tray and bake for about 45 minutes or until tender. Remove from the oven and allow to cool. Scoop out the flesh and purée until smooth using an electric stick blender. If you like you can add a little of your baby's usual milk to thin down the consistency.

nutritional benefits
- *Provides vitamin A*

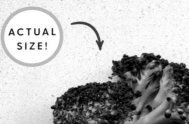

ACTUAL
SIZE!

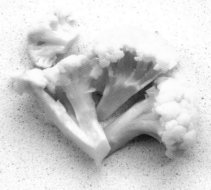

STEAMED BROCCOLI

STEAMED CAULIFLOWER

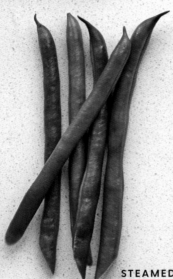

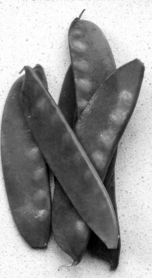

STEAMED GREEN BEANS

STEAMED MANGETOUT

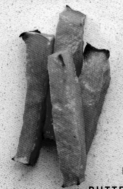

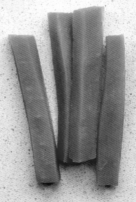

**ROASTED
BUTTERNUT SQUASH**

STEAMED CARROT

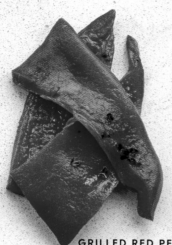

GRILLED RED PEPPER

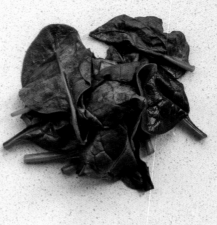

STEAMED SPINACH

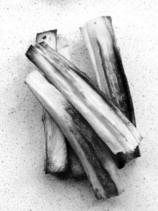

ROASTED PARSNIP

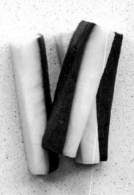

STEAMED COURGETTE

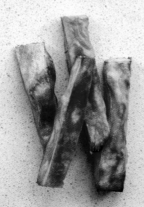

ROASTED SWEET POTATO

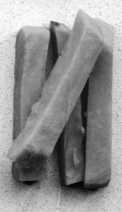

STEAMED SWEET POTATO

SWEET POTATO & POTATO

Finger food

Preheat the oven to 200°C (fan 180°C/gas mark 6). Line a baking tray with baking parchment. Scrub the potato. Cut into wedges approximately 6–7cm long. Spread out in a single layer on the lined tray. Brush with a little sunflower, rapeseed or light olive oil and bake in the oven for 20–25 minutes or until tender.

Purée

Bake

Preheat the oven to 200°C (fan 180°C/gas mark 6). Scrub the potato, prick with a sharp knife. Place on a non-stick baking tray and bake for 45–60 minutes or until tender, depending on size. Remove from the oven, allow to cool down a little. Cut the potato in half, scoop out the flesh and purée in a food processor or with an electric stick blender. You can add a little of your baby's usual milk if you want to thin down the consistency.

Steam

Peel the potato and cut into cubes. Steam for about 12 minutes or until tender. Purée with an electric stick blender or in a food processor adding a little of the water from the bottom of the steamer or some of your baby's usual milk, to make the desired consistency for your baby.

nutritional benefits
- *Sweet potatoes provide vitamin A*
- *A good source of vitamin C*

PARSNIP

Finger food

Bake

Preheat the oven to 200°C (fan 180°C/gas mark 6). Lay a piece of foil on a baking tray, brush with sunflower, rapeseed or light olive oil. Peel and trim small parsnips and cut larger parsnips into pieces about 6–7cm long. Place on the lined tray and brush with oil. Bake for about 15 minutes or until tender.

Steam

Prepare as above and cook in a steamer for about 8 minutes or until tender.

Purée

Steamed parsnip is good mixed with carrot, sweet potato or apple. Purée with an electric stick blender or in a food processor adding a little of the water from the bottom of the steamer or some of your baby's usual milk, to make the desired consistency for your baby.

nutritional benefits
- *Provides vitamin C*

SPINACH

Finger food

Wash a generous handful of baby spinach very carefully. Steam for about 2 minutes or until the leaves are wilted. Gently press out any excess water.

Purée

Steamed spinach is good mixed with root vegetables like carrot, sweet potato or butternut squash. Purée with an electric stick blender or in a food processor adding a little of the water from the bottom of the steamer or some of your baby's usual milk, to make the desired consistency for your baby.

nutritional benefits

- *Provides vitamin A, folate, vitamin C (but losses may occur due to cooking method), iron (see page 40 on absorption), zinc, calcium and some B vitamins*

SWEET RED PEPPER

Finger food

Preheat a grill to high. Cut the red pepper into quarters and grill until the skin has charred. Place in a plastic bag and allow to cool. Peel off the blistered skin and cut the quarters in half for your baby.

Purée

Roasted sweet pepper (see above) is good mixed with vegetables like carrot, sweet potato, butternut squash or cauliflower. Purée with an electric stick blender or in a food processor adding some of your baby's usual milk, to make the desired consistency for your baby.

nutritional benefits

- *Provides vitamin C, A and some B vitamins*

Find images of actual-size finger foods on pp78–9 and the purées on pp82–3

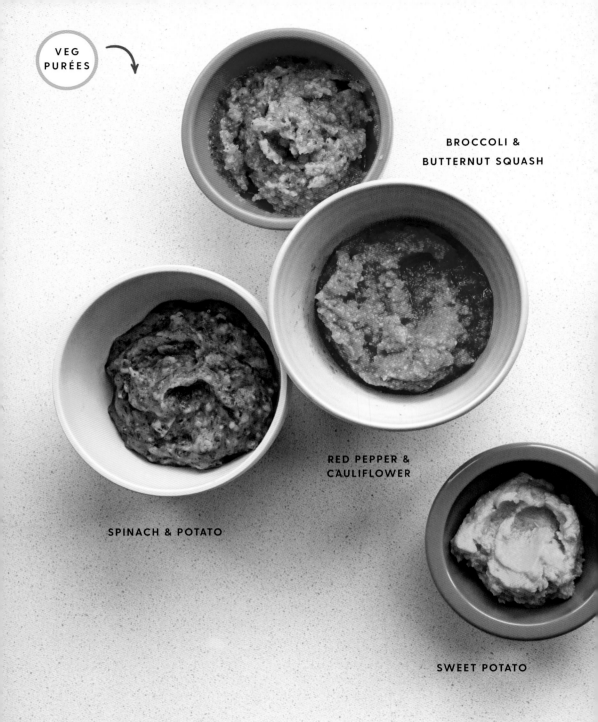

VEG
PURÉES

BROCCOLI &
BUTTERNUT SQUASH

RED PEPPER &
CAULIFLOWER

SPINACH & POTATO

SWEET POTATO

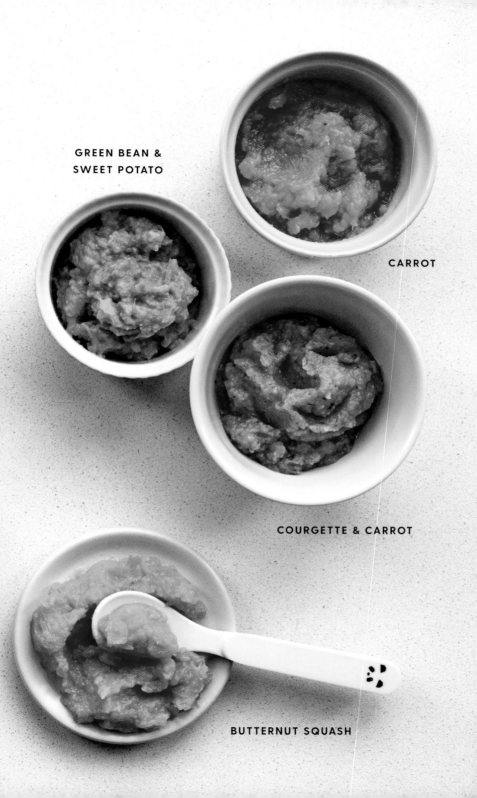

GREEN BEAN &
SWEET POTATO

CARROT

COURGETTE & CARROT

BUTTERNUT SQUASH

fruits

APPLE
Finger food
To begin with raw apple is too hard as a first food so peel the apple, cut it into wedges and steam it for about 3–4 minutes or until tender. For older babies you can try giving wedges of apple with the skin on once they learn to chew.

Purée
Choose a sweet variety of eating apple. Peel, core and dice the apple and put into a heavy based pan with a little water (4-5 tbsp for 2 apples). Cover and cook over a low heat for 6–7 minutes until tender. Purée in a food processor. You can combine with pear or add a little ground cinnamon.

nutritional benefits
- *Provides vitamin C (but losses may occur due to cooking method)*

PEAR
Finger food
For young babies I peel pears and cut them into wedges – just make sure that the pear is soft and ripe. You could try leaving a little skin on the pear to make it easier to hold as they are quite slippery. For older babies wash the pear, leave the skin on and cut into wedges.

Purée
If pears are soft and ripe and your baby is at least 6 months you can simply peel, core and dice the fruit and then blend. Alternatively put peeled, cored and chopped pears into a steamer and steam for 2–3 minutes or until tender. Purée or mash. Pear purée can be quite runny so you may want to mix with mashed banana or puréed apple.

nutritional benefit
- *Provides vitamin C (but losses may occur due to cooking method) and vitamin K*

PEACH
Finger food
I tend to cut peaches into wedges and leave the skin on for finger food, it makes it easier to hold and a lot of the nutrients lie in the skin. Some young babies may find it difficult to digest the skin in which case you can peel the wedges.

Purée
To peel peaches, cut a cross in the base of the peach with a sharp knife. Place them in a pan of boiling water for about 30 seconds. Remove with a slotted spoon and immediately place in a bowl of cold water with ice to cool and stop the cooking process. The skin should peel away easily. Cut the flesh into pieces and mash or blend.

nutritional benefits
- *Provides vitamin C (but losses may occur due to cooking method) and vitamin A*

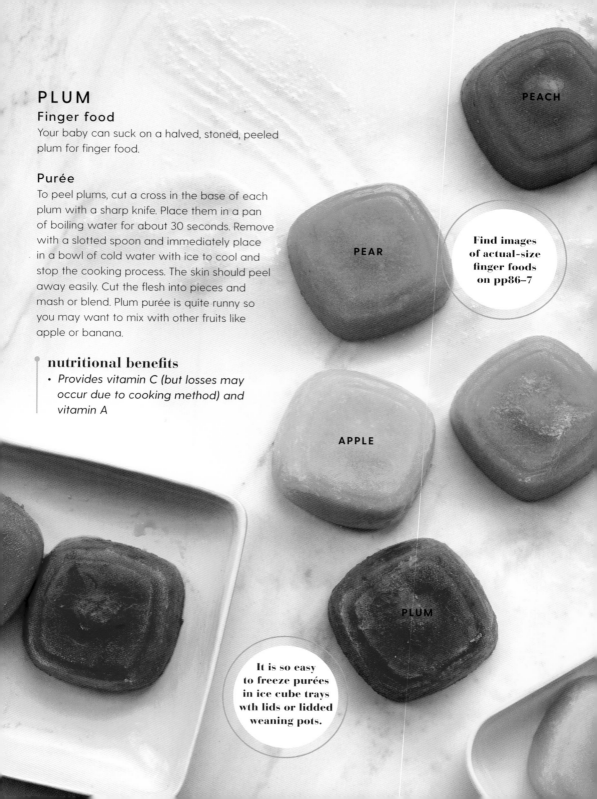

PLUM

Finger food

Your baby can suck on a halved, stoned, peeled plum for finger food.

Purée

To peel plums, cut a cross in the base of each plum with a sharp knife. Place them in a pan of boiling water for about 30 seconds. Remove with a slotted spoon and immediately place in a bowl of cold water with ice to cool and stop the cooking process. The skin should peel away easily. Cut the flesh into pieces and mash or blend. Plum purée is quite runny so you may want to mix with other fruits like apple or banana.

nutritional benefits

- *Provides vitamin C (but losses may occur due to cooking method) and vitamin A*

Find images of actual-size finger foods on pp86–7

It is so easy to freeze purées in ice cube trays wth lids or lidded weaning pots.

PEACH

PEAR

APPLE

PLUM

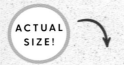

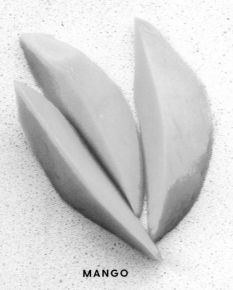

MANGO

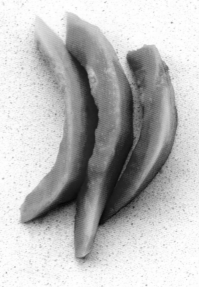

PAPAYA

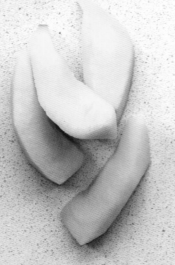

APPLE

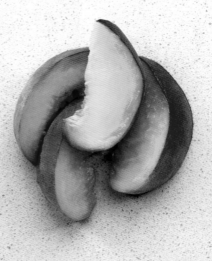

PEACH

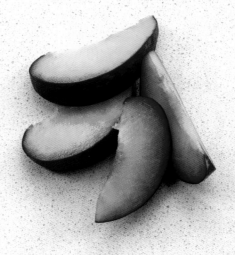

PLUM

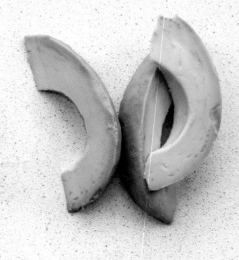

AVOCADO

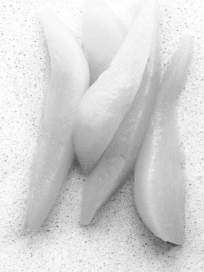

PEAR

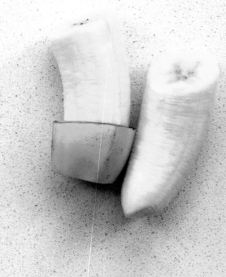

BANANA

no-cook fruits

BANANA
Finger food
Simply peel a small banana and cut into lengths of 6–7cm. As your baby holds food in her fist it needs to be long enough for it to stick out and not too wide, so that she can wrap her fingers around it.

Some babies squeeze the banana and it turns to mush so you may need to leave some of the skin on. Cut a small banana in half and run a knife around the peel about 3cm from the open end. Gently peel back and cut off that strip of peel and give the banana to your baby to hold with the skin on the base.

Purée
Simply mash the banana with a fork until smooth. If it is too thick add a little of your baby's usual milk.

nutritional benefits
- *Provides vitamin B6, vitamin C, magnesium and potassium*

AVOCADO
Finger food
Avocado that isn't over ripe and mushy can also make good finger food. Simply cut the avocado into quarters, peel the skin, then cut the quarters into half again lengthways.

Purée
Cut the avocado in half and remove the stone. Scoop out the flesh into a bowl and mash. A popular combination is mashed avocado and banana.

nutritional benefits
- *Provides vitamin A and a good source of mono-unsaturated fats (similar to olive oil)*

PAPAYA
Finger food
You can try giving papaya wedges to your baby as finger food although it can be mushy.

Purée
Cut a small papaya in half, remove the black seeds and any pith. Scoop the flesh into a bowl and mash. Papaya and banana make a good combination.

nutritional benefits
- *Provides vitamin C and vitamin A*

MANGO
Finger food
Cut peeled mango into wedges.

Purée
Simply mash mango flesh or purée it in a blender. Mango and banana are a good combination.

nutritional benefits
- *Provides vitamin C and vitamin A*

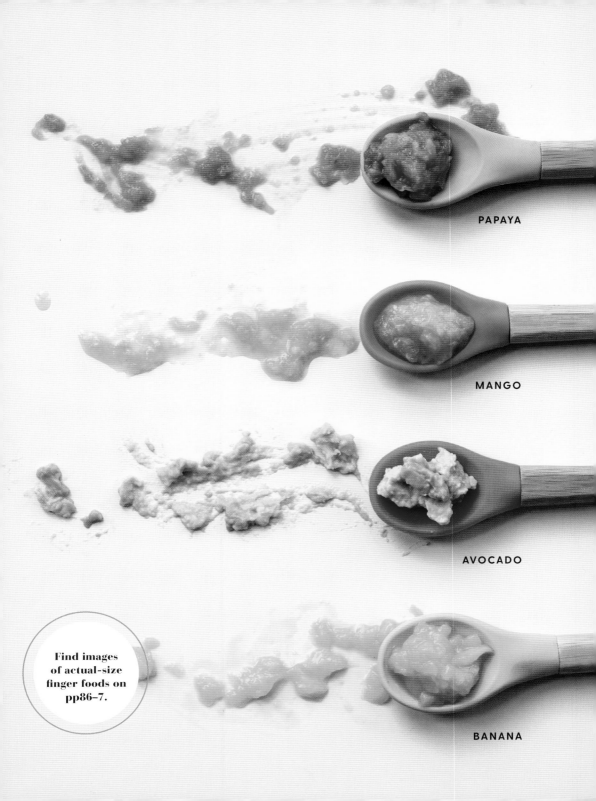

PAPAYA

MANGO

AVOCADO

Find images of actual-size finger foods on pp86–7.

BANANA

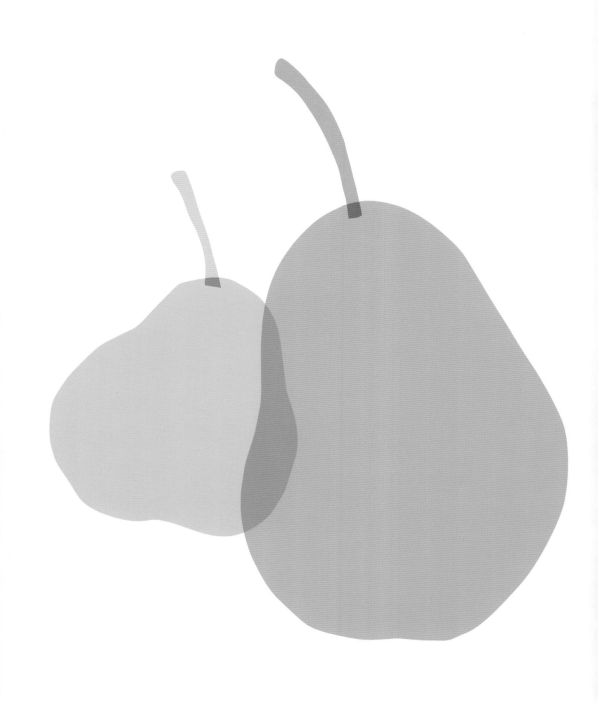

chapter 3

recipes for second stage weaning

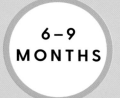

6–9
MONTHS

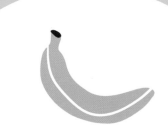

6–9 months
breakfast

weetabix with apple purée

You can't go far wrong with Weetabix! I like to add diced apple for texture and a dose of vitamin C.

makes:
1 portion

1 eating apple, peeled and diced
1 Weetabix
4 tbsp milk

1. Put the apple into a steamer. Steam for 12 minutes until tender. Mash or purée until smooth.

2. Put the Weetabix into a bowl with the milk and mash. Spoon the apple on top of the Weetabix.

nutritional benefits
- *Nutritionally complete*
- *Provides calcium, phosphate, magnesium, iodine, some fat soluble vitamins in milk and vitamin C*
- *Source of prebiotics*

yoghurt, banana & prune

This dish provides a good source of protein which is an essential nutrient for your growing baby.

makes:
1 portion

60g Greek or natural yoghurt
2 ready-to-eat dried prunes, chopped
¼ banana, finely diced
¼ tsp chia seeds

1. Mix together the yoghurt, prunes and banana. Stir well and spoon into a bowl.

2. Sprinkle with chia seeds.

nutritional benefits
- *Good source of protein*
- *Provides calcium, vitamin C, iron (combination increases the absorption of iron) and iodine*

scrambled egg with spinach & tomatoes

This really is the king of breakfasts, placing eggs centre stage! This morning marvel of a dish provides your growing baby with vitamins E, A and C along with calcium and that all-important iron.

makes:
1 portion

a knob of unsalted butter
3 cherry tomatoes, quartered
a handful of spinach

1 egg, beaten
1 tbsp milk
1 tbsp grated Parmesan cheese

1. Put half the butter into a small pan. Add the tomatoes and spinach and fry for a few minutes. Spoon onto a plate.

2. Beat the egg and milk together in a bowl. Melt the remaining butter into the pan, add the egg and stir over a medium heat until scrambled.

3. Add the cooked tomatoes and spinach into the scrambled egg and mix well.

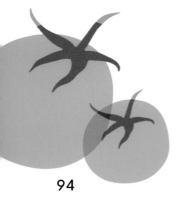

nutritional benefits
- *Nutritionally complete*
- *Provides vitamin E, vitamin A, calcium, vitamin C and iron (combination increases the absorption of iron)*

cheese & chive omelette

It's all in the presentation when it comes to enticing little ones, and simply by cutting an omelette into mini bites or squares, this breakfast staple becomes a finger food win.

makes:
1 portion

1 egg, beaten
1 tbsp milk
1 tbsp grated Cheddar cheese

1 tsp chopped fresh chives
a knob of unsalted butter

1. Mix the egg, milk, cheese and chives together.

2. Heat the butter in a small frying pan. Add the egg mixture. Swirl the pan until most of the mixture is set. Flip the omelette over and cook for another 2–3 minutes, until lightly golden and cooked through.

nutritional benefits
- *Good source of protein*
- *Provides vitamin E, vitamin A, calcium and iodine*

porridge with blueberry, pear & apple

My purple porridge makes for a great start to baby's day. Oats provide a slow release of complex carbs keeping your baby fuelled for longer.

makes:
2 portions

(V)

250ml milk
40g porridge oats
1 eating apple, peeled and grated

1 ripe pear, peeled and diced
75g blueberries

1. Pour the milk into a small pan. Add the oats, apple and pear. Stir over a medium heat until boiling. Simmer for 3 minutes.

2. Add the blueberries and simmer for 2 minutes. Blend until smooth using an electric stick blender.

nutritional benefits

- *Nutritionally complete*
- *Provides calcium, phosphate, magnesium, iodine, some fat-soluble vitamins from the full fat milk and vitamin C*
- *Source of prebiotics*

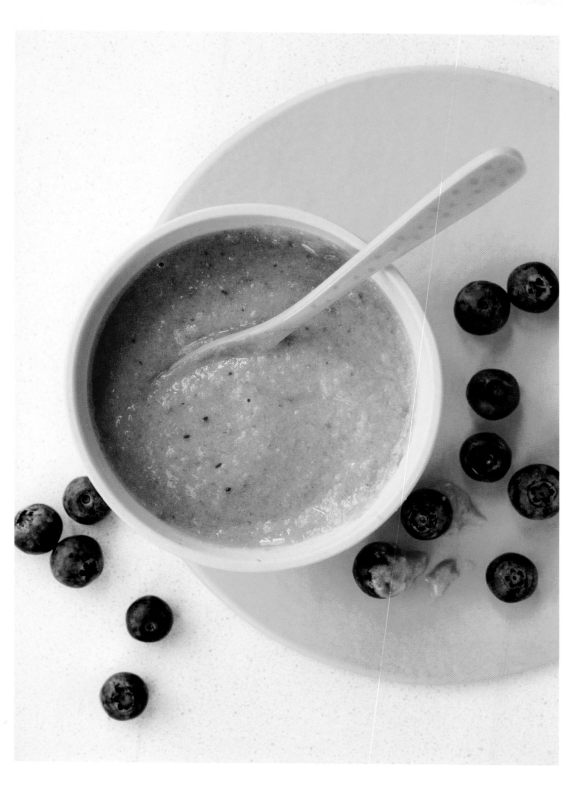

6–9 months
fruit

pear, prune & apple purée

Not only is apple, pear and prune a match made in heaven in the flavour stakes, but prunes can also help to relieve a constipated baby so this is one to remember if your baby is having tummy trouble.

makes:
2 portions

1 ripe pear, peeled and diced
1 eating apple, peeled and diced
3 ready-to-eat dried prunes, diced

1.   Put the pear, apple and prunes into a steamer. Steam for about 8 minutes or until the apple is soft. Purée using an electric stick blender.

nutritional benefits
• *Provides vitamin C*

fruit salad

When starting out you should always take the skin off fruit and many vegetables. The skin introduces a new texture, which can be difficult to manage, and the fibre content is also quite high. So, stick with a simple peeled fruit salad such as this one for a sweet taste of vitamin C and vitamin A for your baby.

makes:
2–3 portions

50g peeled and diced pear
50g peeled and diced papaya or mango
50g peeled and diced cantaloupe melon

1.   Mix all of the diced fruit together in a bowl.

nutritional benefits
• *Provides vitamin C and vitamin A*

99

coconut, apple & strawberry pureé

Shortly after your baby has accepted first tastes you can start to combine foods and flavours. And your baby is sure to approve of this particularly creamy combo.

makes:
2 portions

1 large sweet eating apple, peeled and diced
3 strawberries, hulled and halved
1 small ripe banana, peeled and thickly sliced
2 tbsp full-fat coconut milk

1. Put the diced apple into a steamer and steam for about 6 minutes or until tender.

2. Add the halved strawberries and sliced banana and continue to steam for about 2 minutes or until tender.

3. Purée the steamed fruit and coconut milk using an electric stick blender.

nutritional benefits
- *Provides vitamin C*

coconut, banana & blueberry lollies

Your baby's pearly whites usually start to appear at around 6 months. So, to help soothe their gums make up a batch of these lollies, whatever the weather is doing outside.

makes:
6 lollies

75g ripe banana
75ml full-fat coconut milk
150g blueberries

1. Place all the ingredients in a jug. Blend, using an electric stick blender, until smooth.

2. Pour into six ice lolly moulds.

3. Place in the freezer for 6 hours or until frozen.

nutritional benefits
- *Contains vitamin C, vitamin B*
- *Source of prebiotics*

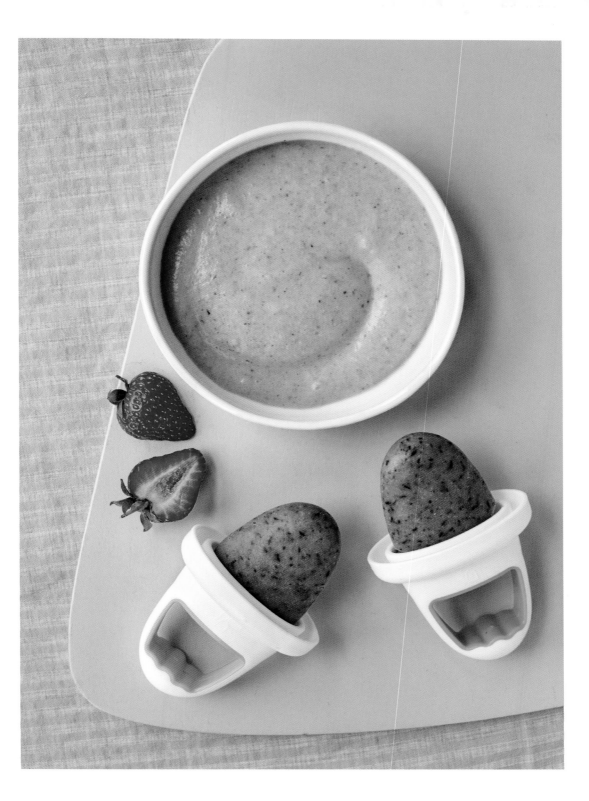

6–9 months
vegetables

roasted vegetables

From 6 months, if your baby is developmentally ready,
you can include soft finger foods on the menu. Roasting
vegetables is a great time-saver too as you can simply
pop everything on a baking tray and roast lots of
different veggies all together while you get on with other
things. Tossing the vegetables in cornflour helps to soak
up some of the excess moisture from them.

makes:
2 portions

1 tbsp olive oil
50g parsnip, peeled and sliced
  into 6cm batons
50g butternut squash, peeled and
  sliced into batons

½ red pepper, sliced into thick
  batons
½ tbsp cornflour

1. Preheat the oven to 200°C (fan 180 °C/gas mark 6). Pour the oil onto
   a baking tray and place in the oven to heat for 5 minutes.

2. Coat the vegetables in the cornflour, then transfer to the baking tray.
   Toss in the oil, to coat, and roast for 20 minutes, to until tender, turning
   halfway through.

nutritional benefits
- *Provides vitamin A, some B vitamins, vitamin C
  and iron (combination increases the absorption of iron)*

103

courgette, pepper, carrot & spinach purée

It's important to pair a vitamin C-rich food with any non-haem (non-meat) iron sources and the good news is that this purée has got both their iron and vitamin C hits covered.

makes:
4 portions

150g carrot, peeled and diced
½ red pepper, diced
1 small eating apple, peeled and diced

200g courgette, sliced
50g spinach

1.   Steam the diced carrot, pepper and apple for 5 minutes.

2.   Add the courgette and steam for a further 4 minutes. Then add the spinach and steam for another 3 minutes.

3.   Purée all the ingredients together, using an electric stick blender, until smooth.

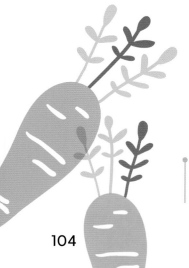

nutritional benefits
• *Provides vitamin A, vitamin C and iron (combination increases the absorption of iron)*

butternut squash & broccoli purée

A purée with a good source of prebiotics can help to keep that gut-friendly bacteria healthy! This simple four-ingredient dish also provides vitamin A, vitamin C and calcium.

makes:
2 portions

200g butternut squash
100g broccoli
40g tomatoes
10g Parmesan cheese, grated

1. Put the squash into a steamer and steam for 8 minutes, add the broccoli and tomatoes and steam for 5 minutes.

2. Purée the butternut squash, broccoli and tomatoes together, using an electric stick blender, to the desired consistency. Stir in the Parmesan cheese.

easy homemade vegetable stock

It is very easy to make your own delicious no-salt vegetable stock, which is suitable for freezing.

makes:
1 litre

1 onion, sliced
4 sticks celery, sliced
1 carrot, peeled and sliced
1 leek, sliced
1 litre of water
3 peppercorns
4 stalks of parsley

1. Put the onion, celery, carrot, leek, water, peppercorns and parsley into a saucepan. Cover with a lid and bring up to the boil. Simmer for 1 hour. Strain through a sieve into a jug or plastic container.

nutritional benefits
- *Provides vitamin A, vitamin C and calcium*
- *Source of prebiotics*

spinach pasta with butternut squash

This is such a tasty and nutritionally balanced meal for your tiny tot. Plus, baby pasta shapes are the perfect size to encourage little ones to learn to chew.

makes:
4 portions

200g butternut squash, cut into 1cm dice
50g baby spinach

50g cream cheese
15g Parmesan cheese, grated
50g baby shell pasta

1. Steam the diced butternut squash for 12 minutes, until just soft. Put half of the squash into a bowl.

2. Put the spinach into a pan and cook, stirring, until wilted. Add the spinach to the squash in the bowl and using an electric stick blender purée until smooth. Pour the vegetable purée into the pan and stir in the cream cheese and Parmesan.

3. Cook the pasta according to the packet instructions. Add the pasta to the sauce with the remaining cooked squash. Stir until well coated.

nutritional benefits
- *Nutritionally complete*
- *Provides vitamin A, vitamin C and calcium*

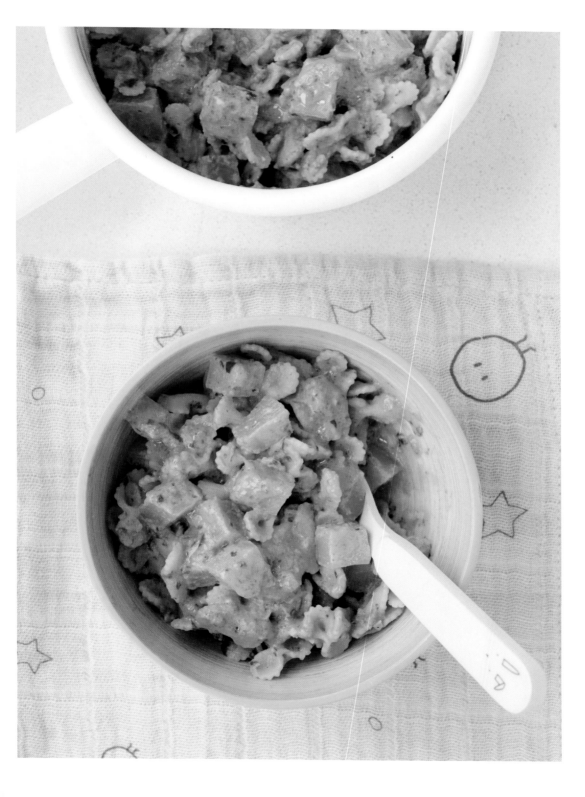

courgette & broccoli frittata

Frittatas will soon be your new go-to! Even on busy days it's easy to rustle up a quick frittata for the whole family, baby included. This has all the nutrients your little one needs from a meal so even if you are pushed for time you can feel confident that their nutritional needs are still covered.

makes:
12 frittata fingers

You will also need:
18cm square
baking tin

butter, for greasing
75g courgettes, cut into
   2cm slices
50g small broccoli florets
3 eggs
1 tbsp milk
20g Cheddar cheese, grated
20g Parmesan cheese, grated
2 tbsp chopped fresh basil

1. Grease the tin lightly with butter. Steam the courgette and broccoli for 3-4 minutes until tender. Cool and roughly chop.

2. Beat the eggs, milk, cheeses and basil together in a bowl. Add the vegetables and stir.

3. Pour the mixture into the tin and bake for 15 minutes or until firm and set in the middle.

4. Allow to cool slightly, then remove from the tin and slice into twelve fingers.

nutritional benefits
- *Nutritionally complete*
- *Provides vitamin A, vitamin E, calcium, vitamin C and iron (combination increases the absorption of iron)*

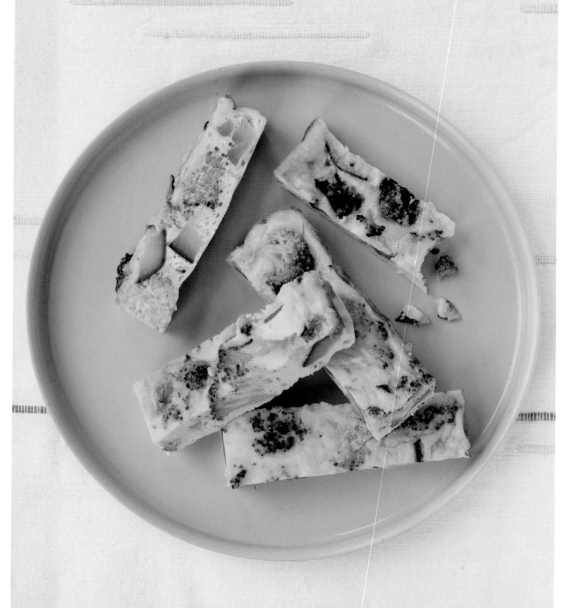

tomato & butternut squash pasta

This tomato and butternut squash sauce is delicious paired with orzo pasta, which has a nice soft texture that's ideal for weaning babies.

makes:
3 portions

100g butternut squash, peeled and cut into 1cm dice
10g unsalted butter

3 tomatoes, skinned, deseeded and chopped
4 basil leaves, chopped
25g orzo pasta

1. Steam the squash for 12 minutes or until soft. Blend until smooth using an electric stick blender.

2. Melt the butter in a small pan. Add the chopped tomatoes and stir over the heat until soft. Add the basil and squash purée.

3. Cook the pasta according to the packet instructions. Drain, reserving 1 tablespoon of the cooking water. Add the pasta and cooking water to the sauce and stir to combine.

nutritional benefits
- *Provides vitamin A, vitamin C*

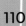

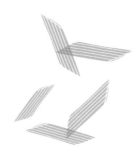

carrot, sweet potato & lentils with pasta

Root vegetables such as sweet potato and carrot are always a firm favourite with babies and using a flavour they are familiar with (and enjoy) can encourage them to try new textures such as the lentils and pasta here.

makes:
4 portions

1 tsp sunflower oil
½ onion, chopped
100g carrot, thinly sliced
200g sweet potato, peeled and
 cut into 1cm dice
20g red lentils

300ml homemade vegetable stock
 (see page 105), very low-salt
 vegetable stock or water
1 tsp tomato purée
15g baby pasta (25g cooked
 weight)

1. Heat the oil in a pan. Add the onion and fry for 2 minutes. Add the carrot, sweet potato, red lentils, stock and tomato purée.

2. Stir to combine, then cover and simmer for 20 minutes, until the vegetables are tender.

3. Meanwhile, cook the baby pasta according to the packet instructions. Drain and set aside.

4. Purée the cooked vegetable mixture, to the desired consistency, using an electric stick blender.

5. Add the cooked baby pasta to the purée and stir to combine.

nutritional benefits
- *Nutritionally complete*
- *Provides vitamin A, vitamin C*
- *Source of prebiotics*

quinoa with mediterranean vegetables

It's time to take baby on a food adventure with a quick and tasty trip to the Med! Quinoa is a great ingredient to use as an alternative to rice or pasta and when paired with Mediterranean flavours including tomato, red pepper, courgette, basil and garlic your baby will be exposed to new tastes, textures and nutrients, too.

makes:
2 portions

25g quinoa
2 tsp sunflower oil
30g onion, finely diced
30g red pepper, finely diced
30g courgette, finely diced

30g carrot, peeled and finely diced
½ clove garlic, crushed
6 cherry tomatoes, diced
1 tbsp chopped fresh basil

1. Cook the quinoa according to the packet instructions. Drain and set aside.

2. Heat the oil in a pan. Add the onion, pepper, courgette and carrot. Fry for 5 minutes.

3. Add the garlic and tomatoes, fry for 2 minutes, then add the cooked quinoa and basil. Stir to combine.

nutritional benefits
- *Nutritionally complete*
- *Provides vitamin A, vitamin C and iron (combination increases the absorption of iron)*

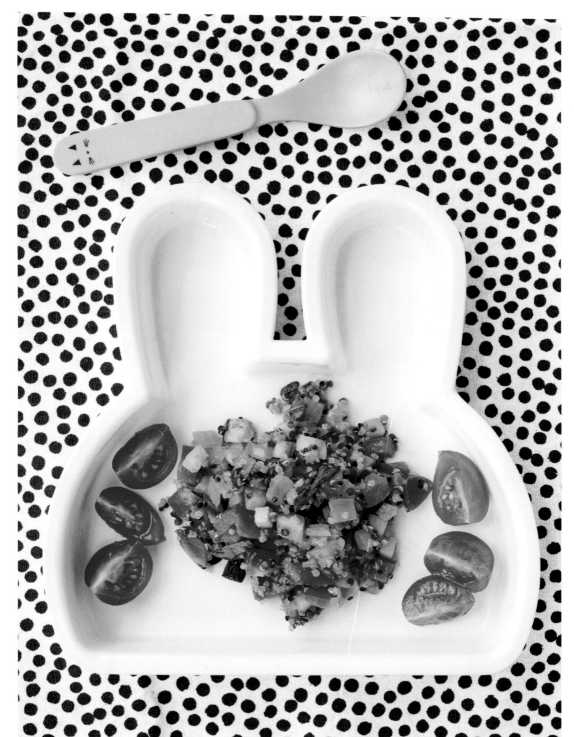

2-IN-1 RECIPE

It's good to offer a mix of purées and soft finger foods, so here's a variation on the same recipe. Your baby can have a purée one day and finger food the next. After all, variety is the spice of life!

FINGER FOOD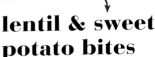

lentil & sweet potato bites

makes:
12 bites

1 x 200g sweet potato, scrubbed
70g cooked Puy lentils
1 small onion, finely sliced
40g baby spinach
25g Parmesan cheese, grated
olive oil, for drizzling

1. Prick the sweet potato with a sharp knife. Cook the whole potato in the microwave for 8 minutes or until soft. Leave to cool. When cold, scoop out the flesh.

2. Put the potato flesh, lentils, spring onions, spinach and cheese in a food processor. Whiz until finely chopped.

3. Preheat the oven to 220°C (fan 200°C/ gas mark 7). Line a baking tray with baking parchment.

4. Shape the mixture into twelve small bites and place on the lined tray. Drizzle with oil and roll to coat. Bake for 15 minutes until lightly golden. Leave on the tray for 5 minutes before removing, to cool. You can allow to cool and freeze.

THE PURÉE

lentil & sweet potato purée

makes:
6 portions

Same ingredients as listed left
with the addition of:
200ml homemade vegetable stock (see page 105) or very low-salt vegetable stock

1. Cook the sweet potato as per step 1 in the bites recipe (see left).

2. Heat 1 teaspoon olive oil in a pan. Add the onion and fry for 2 minutes. Add the potato flesh, lentils and stock. Cover and simmer for 15 minutes until soft. Add the spinach and allow to cook for 15 seconds, then remove from the heat and mash or whiz to the desired consistency.

nutritional benefits of both

- *Nutritionally complete*
- *Provides vitamin A, vitamin C, iron (combination increases the absorption or iron) and zinc*
- *Source of prebiotics*

lentil, kale & carrot purée

Simple but nutritionally supercharged, this purée provides your baby with vitamin A, vitamin C, iron and zinc.

makes:
3–4 portions

1 tsp sunflower oil
½ red onion, chopped
100g carrot, peeled and sliced
40g red lentils
250ml homemade vegetable stock (see page 105) or very low-salt vegetable stock
30g kale, chopped

1. Heat the oil in a pan. Add the onion and carrot and fry for 2–3 minutes. Add the lentils and stock and simmer for 15 minutes.

2. Add the kale and simmer for another 5 minutes until tender. Blend to the desired consistency using an electric stick blender.

nutritional benefits
- *Nutritionally complete*
- *Provides vitamin A, vitamin C, iron (combination increases the absorption of iron) and zinc*
- *Source of prebiotics*

sweet potato, parsnip & spinach purée

Steaming is one of the best ways to prepare dishes because it helps fruit and veg retain its levels of water-soluble vitamins such as vitamin C.

makes:
4 portion

250g sweet potatoes, peeled and cut into 1cm dice
100g parsnip, peeled and cut into 1cm dice
1 tbsp olive oil (optional)
75g baby spinach

1. Steam the diced sweet potato and parsnip for 12 minutes, until just soft. Alternatively preheat the oven to 200°C (fan 180 °C/gas mark 6), toss the diced veg in 1 tablespoon olive oil and roast in the oven for approximately 20 minutes, turning halfway through.

2. Steam the spinach for 3 minutes. Then transfer to a blender with the steamed or roasted veg and purée until smooth.

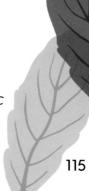

nutritional benefits
- *Provides vitamins A and C*
- *Provides iron*

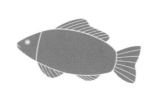

6–9 months
fish

salmon, dill & sweet potato bites

Salmon with dill is such a classic flavour combination and using herbs is a great way to add seasoning and depth of flavour to your baby's dishes without the need for salt.

makes:
12 bites

1 x 200g sweet potato
4 spring onions, sliced
30g Parmesan cheese, grated
a squeeze of lemon juice
2 tbsp chopped fresh dill

200g salmon fillet, skinned
   and diced
40g panko breadcrumbs
sunflower oil, for frying

1. Scrub and prick the potato with a sharp knife. Cook the whole potato in the microwave for 8 minutes or until soft. Alternatively preheat the oven to 200°C (fan 180°C/gas mark 6), and roast the sweet potato in the oven for approximately 50 minutes until tender. Leave to cool. When cold, scoop out the flesh.

2. Put the cooked sweet potato flesh, spring onions, Parmesan, lemon, salmon, dill and half of the breadcrumbs into a food processor. Whiz until the mixture has come together.

3. Shape into twelve sausage shapes and roll in the remaining breadcrumbs.

4. Heat a little oil in a large non-stick frying pan. Pan-fry the bites for 10–12 minutes over a medium heat until golden and cooked through.

nutritional benefits
- *Good source of protein*
- *Provides omega 3s, vitamin A, vitamin C, iron (combination increases the absorption of iron), calcium and zinc*

2-IN-1 RECIPE Nutritionally speaking, salmon and broccoli are two food heroes. And because this such an all-round recipe I have created two versions, the purée and a finger food version – you are welcome!

THE PURÉE

salmon & broccoli purée

makes:
4 portions

2 tsp sunflower oil
200g potato, peeled and chopped
2 spring onions
200ml homemade vegetable stock (see
  page 105) or very low-salt vegetable stock
150g broccoli florets
120g salmon fillet, diced
25g Parmesan, grated
3 tbsp milk

1. Heat 2 teaspoons of oil in a pan. Add the potato and spring onions and fry for 2 minutes. Add the stock. Cover with a lid and simmer for 10–12 minutes.

2 Add the broccoli and salmon, cover and simmer for 5–6 minutes until tender. Stir in the cheese and milk and blend or mash to the desired consistency.

nutritional benefits of both

- *Nutritionally complete*
- *Provides omega 3s, vitamin A, vitamin C, calcium, iron and zinc*
- *Source of prebiotics*

FINGER FOOD

salmon & broccoli croquettes

makes:
10 croquettes

Same ingredients as listed left minus the stock and raw potato and with the addition of:
150g cold mashed potato (cooked without salt
  in the water)
50g panko breadcrumbs
1 egg, beaten
1 tbsp sunflower oil

1. Preheat the oven to 200°C (fan 180°C/ gas mark 6). Cook the broccoli in boiling water for 5 minutes. Drain and chop.

2. Bake the salmon, wrapped in foil, in the oven for 12 minutes or until cooked. Flake the fish and leave to cool, then mix together with the potato, spring onions, broccoli, half the breadcrumbs, the cheese and egg. Shape into ten croquettes and roll in the remaining breadcrumbs. Chill for 30 minutes.

3. Heat the oil in a frying pan. Add the croquettes. Fry for 5–8 minutes until golden and crisp. You can also allow to cool and freeze.

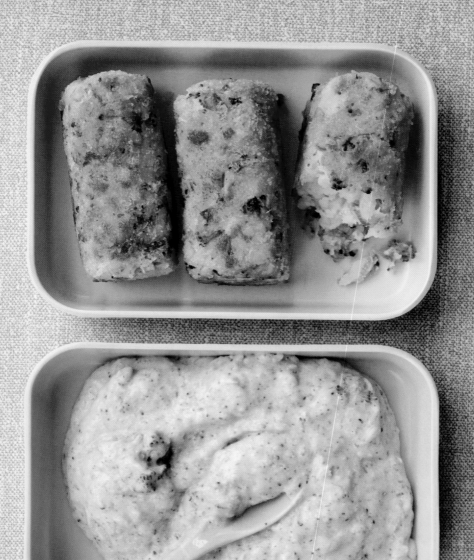

salmon, sweet potato & spinach purée

The sooner you can establish oily fish on your tot's menu the better. Salmon and sweet potato is such a fantastic flavour combination.

makes:
3 portions

a knob of unsalted butter
100g sweet potatoes, peeled and diced
100g tomatoes, chopped
115g salmon fillet, skinned, all bones removed and diced
30g spinach
10g Cheddar cheese, grated

1. Melt the butter in a pan and stir in the sweet potato. Add the tomatoes and 100ml water. Cover and simmer for 12 minutes or until soft.

2. Add the salmon and spinach and cook for another 3–4 minutes, until cooked through. Stir in the cheese and mash or blend to the desired consistency.

nutritional benefits
- *Provides vitamin A, vitamin C, iodine, calcium, iron and zinc*

tuna, pepper & squash purée

This nutritious all-in-one dish is full of vibrant veggies to make it not only taste good but look good too.

makes:
4 portions

1 tbsp olive oil
2 spring onions, chopped
175g potatoes, peeled and cut into 1cm dice
140g butternut squash, peeled and cut into 1cm dice
50g red pepper, peeled and cut into 1cm dice
400g tin chopped tomatoes
40g tinned sweetcorn
50g tuna in sunflower oil, drained
1 tbsp chopped fresh basil
20g Parmesan cheese, grated

1. Heat the oil in a pan. Add the onions, potatoes, squash and pepper. Fry for 2 minutes. Add the tomatoes, corn and tuna, cover and simmer for 15 minutes.

3   Stir in the basil and Parmesan and mash or blend to the desired consistency.

nutritional benefits
- *Nutritionally complete*
- *Provides vitamin A, vitamin C, B vitamins, calcium, magnesium, iodine, iron and zinc*
- *Source of prebiotics*

2-IN-1 RECIPE

This tasty recipe can be made two ways using mostly the same ingredients. Whether it's served as a purée or a burger it certainly delivers a powerful trio of superfoods for your baby.

THE PURÉE

salmon & kale purée

makes:
3 portions

175g butternut squash, peeled
25g kale
120g salmon fillet, skinned, all bones removed
  and sliced into pieces
25g Parmesan cheese, grated
a squeeze of lemon juice

1. Cube the butternut squash and steam it for 10 minutes. Add the kale and salmon to the steamer and steam for another 5 minutes until cooked through. Put everything into a bowl.

2. Stir in 2 tablespoons of water, the Parmesan and lemon juice. Blend until smooth using an electric stick blender.

nutritional benefits
- *Provides omega 3s, vitamin A, vitamin C, calcium, iodine, iron and zinc*

FINGER FOOD

salmon & kale burgers

makes:
8 portions

Same ingredients as listed left
with the addition of:
3 spring onions, sliced
25g panko breadcrumbs
plain flour, for coating
sunflower oil, for frying

1. Grate the butternut squash and put with all of the ingredients, except the flour, into a food processor. Whiz until finely chopped. Shape into eight equal-sized burgers.

2. Coat the burgers in plain flour. Heat a little oil in a large non-stick frying pan. Fry the burgers for 3–4 minutes on each side until lightly golden and cooked through. You can also allow to cool and freeze once cooked.

nutritional benefits
- *Provides omega 3s, vitamin A, vitamin C, calcium, iodine, iron and zinc*
- *Source of prebiotics*

salmon in tomato sauce with baby pasta shells

It is so important to include oily fish like salmon in your baby's diet, ideally twice a week, as it contains essential fatty acids that are vital for brain and visual development. The addition of carrot, tomato, apple and Parmesan here will encourage little ones to give fish a try if they weren't too sure before.

makes:
4 portions

1 tbsp olive oil
1 small onion, chopped
1 small carrot, peeled and grated
½ eating apple, peeled and grated
1 clove garlic, crushed

250ml passata
40g baby pasta shells
100g cooked salmon fillet, all bones removed and flaked
1 tbsp grated Parmesan cheese

1. Heat the oil in a pan. Add the onion, carrot and apple and fry for 3–4 minutes. Add the garlic and fry for 30 seconds. Add the passata. Cover and simmer for 10 minutes.

2. Cook the pasta according to the packet instructions. Drain.

3. Stir the drained pasta into the sauce with the flaked salmon and cheese. If you prefer you can blend the sauce, then mix with the pasta and flaked salmon.

nutritional benefits
- *Good source of protein*
- *Provides omega 3s, vitamin A, vitamin C, iron (combination increases the absorption of iron) calcium, iodine and zinc*
- *Source of prebiotics*

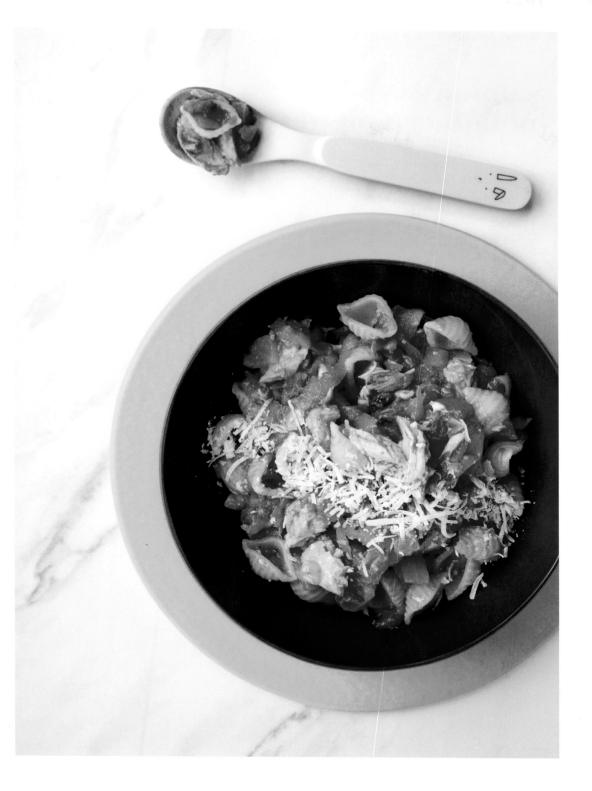

salmon & sweet potato croquettes

Whether it's a leisurely picnic in the park or a swift lunch on the go, these croquettes will live up to baby's expectations! They are also suitable for freezing once cooked so make extra if you have time and simply defrost overnight in the fridge, then reheat in the oven.

makes:
15 croquettes

1 x 250g sweet potato
130g butternut squash, peeled and grated
30g red onion, finely chopped
50g tinned sweetcorn
200g salmon fillet, skinned, all
bones removed and diced
30g Cheddar cheese, grated
a squeeze of lemon juice
1 tomato, deseeded and chopped
40g panko breadcrumbs
sunflower oil, for frying

1. Scrub and prick the potato with a sharp knife. Cook the whole potato in the microwave for 8 minutes or until soft. Alternatively preheat the oven to 200°C (fan 180°C/gas mark 6), and roast the sweet potato in the oven for approximately 50 minutes until tender. Leave to cool. When cold, scoop out the flesh.

2. Put the potato flesh into a food processor with the vegetables, salmon, cheese, lemon juice, tomato and 40g breadcrumbs. Blitz the ingredients for a few seconds, until well combined.

3. Shape the mixture into fifteen croquettes and coat in the remaining breadcrumbs. Heat the oil in a large non-stick frying pan and fry the croquettes for 8–10 minutes or until cooked through.

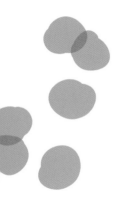

nutritional benefits
- *Provides omega 3s, vitamin A, vitamin C, iron (combination increases the absorption of iron) calcium, iodine and zinc*
- *Source of prebiotics*

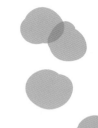

cod & couscous balls

I love this recipe, which you can make ahead and freeze once cooked. It's fantastic for those who have a fussy eater as it lets baby exercise their independent side. The balls are packed full of essential nutrients making it a nutritionally complete mouthful, so mum and dad are happy too.

makes:
20 balls

100g cooked couscous (or 40g uncooked weight)
120g cod fillet, all bones removed
4 spring onions, sliced
1 small carrot, peeled and grated
½ eating apple, peeled and grated
40g Parmesan cheese, grated
2 tbsp fresh basil, chopped
1 egg yolk
sunflower oil, for drizzling

1. If you're using uncooked couscous, cook it according to packet instructions and leave to cool slightly. Preheat the oven to 200°C (fan 180°C/gas mark 6). Line a baking tray with baking parchment.

2. Place all the ingredients, except the egg yolk, into a food processor. Whiz until finely chopped, then stir through the egg yolk. Shape into twenty balls.

3. Place the balls on the lined tray and drizzle with a little oil. Bake for 20 minutes, turning over once, halfway through the cooking time.

nutritional benefits
- *Nutritionally complete*
- *Provides vitamin A, vitamin C, vitamin E, iodine, calcium, iron and zinc*
- *Source of prebiotics*

cod, spinach, potato & pea purée

Oily fish such as salmon is essential as it contains those all-important omega 3s in your baby's diet. However, you can also add white fish to your mealtime repertoire as it's a great source of protein and iron and this cod purée is one of my favourites.

makes:
6 portions

a knob of butter
1 small leek, sliced
1 small carrot, peeled and cut into 1.5cm dice
1 medium potato, peeled and cut into 1.5cm dice
2 tbsp plain flour
200ml homemade vegetable stock (see page 105) or very low-salt vegetable stock
50g cod loin, skinned, all bones removed and diced
30g frozen peas
30g baby spinach
100ml milk
2 tbsp grated Parmesan cheese

1. Melt the butter in a pan. Add the leek and carrot and fry for 3 minutes. Add the potato and flour and gradually stir in the stock. Bring to the boil, cover and simmer for 10 minutes.

2. Add the cod, peas, spinach and milk to the pan. Simmer for 5 minutes until the mixture is soft and the cod is cooked. Remove from the heat and stir in the cheese.

3. Purée or mash to the desired consistency.

nutritional benefits
- *Good source of protein*
- *Provides vitamin A, vitamin C, zinc (combination increases the absorption of iron) calcium, iodine*
- *Source of prebiotics*

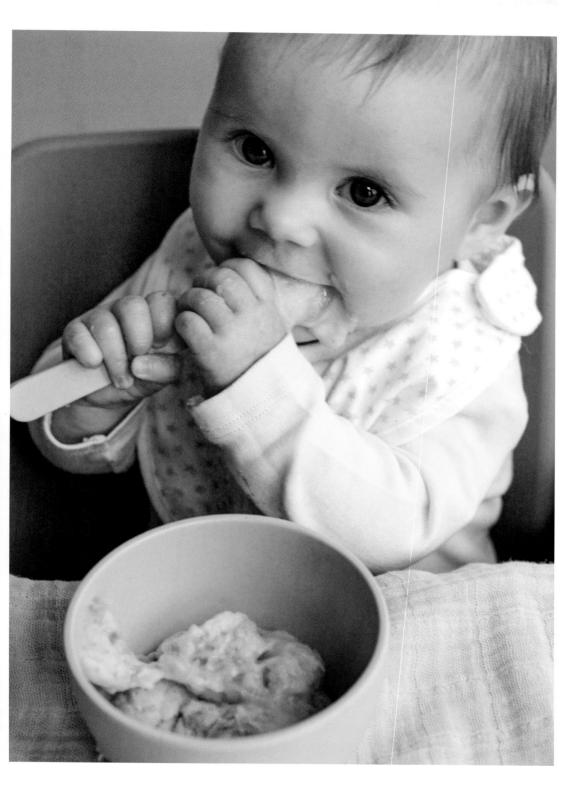

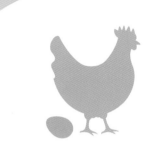

6–9 months
poultry

mini chicken pies

By using half the quantity of chicken casserole with squash (see page 138) you can quickly cook up a whole new dish with my baby-friendly mini chicken pies.

If you just want to make chicken pies then use the full amount of the chicken casserole recipe and double the potato topping, below.

makes:
2 pies

....

You will also need
2 x 10cm diameter,
5cm deep ramekins
(*or 3 smaller ramekins
if you prefer*)

300g potatoes, peeled and diced
a small knob of unsalted butter
30g Cheddar cheese, grated

2 tbsp milk
½ quantity chicken casserole with
    butternut squash (see page 138)

1. Preheat the oven to 220°C (fan 200°C/gas mark 7).

2. Bring a pan of water to the boil, add the diced potatoes and boil for 10–12 minutes or until tender. Drain, mash and mix with the butter, cheese and milk.

3. Spoon the chicken casserole into the ramekins and top with the mash, spreading it out to cover the filling. Bake for 15 minutes.

nutritional benefits
· *Nutritionally complete*
· *Provides vitamin A, vitamin C, iron (combination increases the absorption of iron) calcium and zinc*
· *Source of prebiotics*

my first chicken curry

Some parents are surprised to hear that their baby can enjoy a tasty curry from so early on in their weaning journey. Once your little one is around 7–8 months old, they will probably like a mild, aromatic chicken curry (and you will too!).

makes:
4 portions

1 tbsp olive oil
½ onion, sliced
½ red pepper, deseeded and cut into 1cm dice
200g butternut squash, peeled and cut into 1cm dice
200g chicken thigh fillet, cut into 1.5cm dice

½ tsp mild korma curry powder
½ tsp grated fresh ginger
175ml homemade chicken stock (see page 142), very low-salt chicken stock or water
3 dried apricots, finely chopped
rice, to serve (*optional*)

1. Heat the oil in a pan. Add the onion, pepper, squash and chicken. Brown over the heat for 2 minutes.

2. Add the curry powder and ginger and fry for 30 seconds.

3. Add the stock and apricots. Bring to the boil then cover and simmer for 20 minutes.

4. Blend to a chunky or smooth consistency. Serve with rice, if liked.

nutritional benefits
- *Good source of protein and if served with rice a nutritionally complete meal*
- *Provides vitamin A, iron and zinc*
- *Source of prebiotics*

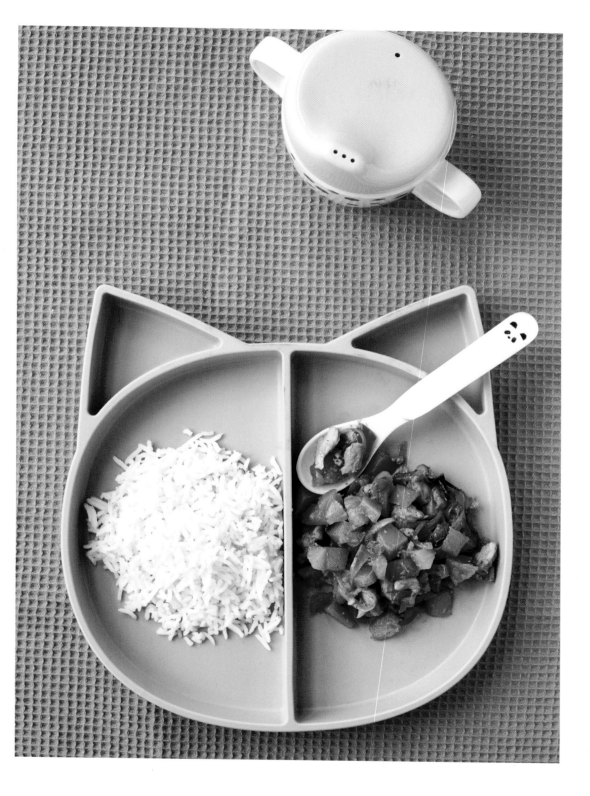

chicken with apricots

There's nothing like the flavour, colour and natural sweetness of fruit to encourage little ones to lap up meals. This protein-packed fruity flavour combination is sure to be a hit.

makes:
4 portions

2 tsp light olive oil
1 small onion, chopped
1 small clove garlic, crushed
75g chicken breast or thigh fillet, cut into 1.5cm dice
3 dried apricots, finely chopped

150g sweet potato, peeled and cut into 1.5cm dice
330ml passata
150ml homemade chicken stock (see page 142), very low-salt chicken stock or water

1. Heat the oil in a pan and sauté the onion for about 5 minutes or until softened.

2. Add the garlic and cook for 1 minute. Add the chicken and sauté for 2–3 minutes.

3. Add the apricots, sweet potato, passata and stock. Bring to the boil then cover and simmer for about 15 minutes. Finely chop or blend to the desired consistency.

nutritional benefits
- *Good source of protein*
- *Provides vitamin A, vitamin C, iron (combination increases the absorption of iron) zinc, calcium*
- *Source of prebiotics*

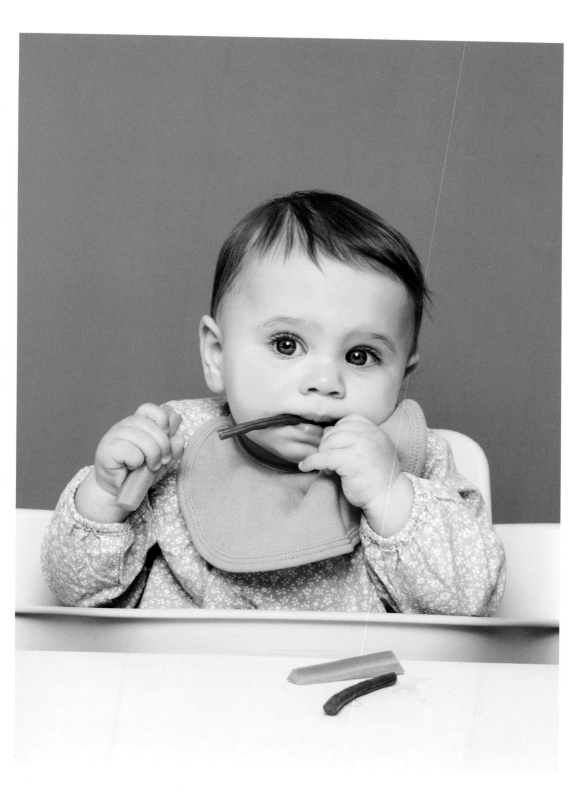

2-IN-1 RECIPE

Baby's first Christmas is such a magical time for everyone. Your little elf will make light work of my turkey balls and my turkey purée – using the same ingredients but served in two ways.

FINGER FOOD

turkey meatballs

makes:
25 balls

1 x 150g sweet potato
75g parsnip, peeled
1 onion, chopped
200g minced turkey thigh
30g spinach
20g Cheddar cheese, grated
1 tsp chopped fresh thyme
30g panko breadcrumbs
2 tsp sunflower oil

1. Scrub and prick the potato with a sharp knife. Cook the whole potato in the microwave for 8 minutes or until soft. Leave to cool. When cold, scoop out the flesh. Grate the parsnip.

2. Place the potato flesh and all the remaining ingredients, except the oil, into a food processor. Whiz until finely chopped. Shape the mixture into 25 balls.

3. Heat the oil in a frying pan. Fry the balls for 8–10 minutes, turning until golden and cooked through. Alternatively preheat the oven to 180°C (fan 160°C/gas mark 4) and cook the balls for about 15 minutes, turning halfway through. You can allow to cool and freeze once cooked.

THE PURÉE

turkey purée

makes:
4 portions

Same ingredients as listed left without the breadcrumbs and with the addition of:
200ml homemade chicken stock (see page 142), very low-salt chicken stock or water

1. Peel and dice the sweet potato and parsnip. Heat the oil in a pan. Add the onion and fry for 3 minutes.

2. Add the parsnip, sweet potato and turkey and brown for 3 minutes. Add the stock, cover and simmer for 15 minutes.

3. Add the spinach and thyme and stir until the spinach has wilted. Blend to the desired consistency then stir in the cheese.

nutritional benefits of both

- *Good source of protein*
- *Provides vitamin A, vitamin C, iron (combination increases the absorption of iron) calcium, selenium and zinc*

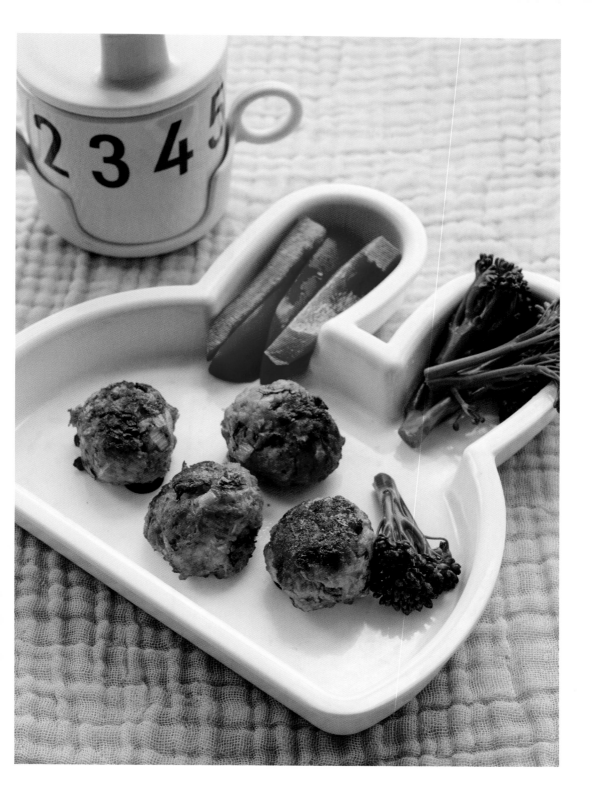

2-IN-1 RECIPE

Two for the price of one! Transform my chicken, quinoa, apple & sage balls into a smooth or textured purée. I love cooking with sage as it adds real depth of flavour to recipes.

FINGER FOOD

chicken, quinoa, apple & sage balls

makes:
25 balls

250g chicken thigh, diced
1 onion, diced
1 eating apple, peeled and diced
1 small carrot, peeled and grated
1 clove garlic, crushed
70g cooked quinoa
2 tbsp chopped fresh sage
40g Parmesan cheese, grated
40g panko breadcrumbs
oil, for frying

1. Place all the ingredients, except the oil, into a food processor. Whiz until the mixture has come together. Shape into twenty-five balls.

2. Heat a little oil in a large frying pan. Fry the balls for 10–12 minutes until golden brown and cooked through. You can allow to cool and freeze once cooked.

THE PURÉE

chicken, quinoa, apple & sage purée

makes:
5 portions

Same ingredients as listed left without the breadcrumbs and with the addition of:
300ml homemade chicken stock (see page 142), very low-salt chicken stock or water

1. Heat 2 teaspoons of oil in a pan. Add the chicken, onion, apple, carrot and garlic and fry for 3–4 minutes.

2. Blend in the stock. Add the quinoa, stir and simmer for 15 minutes.

3. Stir in the sage and Parmesan and blend to the desired consistency.

nutritional benefits of both
- *Good source of protein*
- *Provides vitamin A, vitamin C, iron (combination increases iron absorption), zinc, calcium*
- *Source of prebiotics*

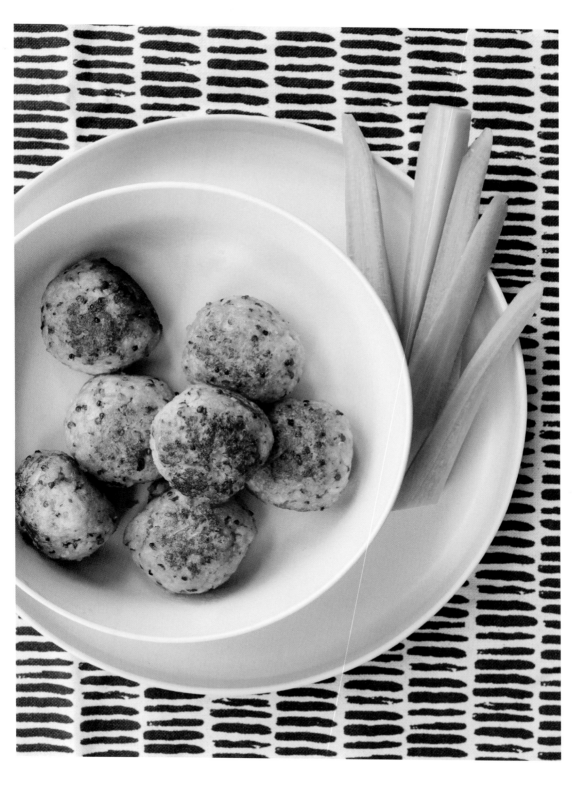

chicken casserole with butternut squash

You can't beat a homemade chicken casserole and this one is sure to satisfy hungry little tums. Either blend or mash to the desired consistency and serve with rice if you wish. This is also a great example of where you can scale the recipe up and serve as a dish for the whole family.

makes:
3 portions

30g unsalted butter
1 leek, chopped
100g butternut squash, peeled and cut into 1.5cm dice
1 clove garlic, crushed
3 tbsp plain flour
200ml homemade chicken stock (see page 142), very low-salt
chicken stock or water
200ml milk
200g chicken breast, cut into 1.5cm dice
1 tsp fresh thyme, chopped
3 tbsp grated Parmesan cheese
rice, to serve (*optional*)

1. Melt the butter in a pan. Add the leek and squash and fry for 4–5 minutes. Add the garlic and fry for 30 seconds. Add the flour, then blend in the stock. Stir until thickened and boiling and the vegetables are tender.

2. Add the milk and bring up to the boil. Add the chicken, cover and simmer for 5 minutes or until the chicken is cooked through. Add the thyme and Parmesan. Serve with rice, if liked.

nutritional benefits

- *Provides vitamin A, vitamin C, iron (combination increases the absorption of iron), calcium and zinc*
- *Source of prebiotics*

2-IN-1 RECIPE

Chicken is often a favourite with babies, which is great news as it is incredibly nutritious, containing high levels of zinc and iron. These recipes include similar ingredients, served in two different ways.

FINGER FOOD

chicken & pea croquettes

makes:
10 croquettes

150g cold mashed potato (cooked without salt in the water)
2 spring onions, sliced
25g Parmesan cheese, grated
40g butternut squash, peeled and grated
75g cooked chicken, diced
40g cooked peas
1 tsp chopped fresh thyme
1 egg, beaten
50g panko breadcrumbs
2 tbsp oil

1. Place the potato, spring onions, Parmesan, butternut squash, chicken and peas into a bowl with the egg and thyme. Mix well and shape into ten croquettes.

2. Roll in the breadcrumbs. Heat 2 tablespoons of oil in a frying pan. Fry the croquettes for 5–8 minutes, on each side, until golden and heated through. You can allow to cool and freeze once cooked.

THE PURÉE

chicken & pea purée

makes:
4 portions

a knob of unsalted butter
2 spring onions, sliced
175g potatoes, peeled and diced
1 tbsp chopped fresh thyme
75g butternut squash, peeled and diced
200ml homemade chicken stock (see page 142), very low-salt chicken stock or water
50g peas
100g cooked chicken, diced
25g Parmesan cheese, grated

1. Melt the butter in a pan. Add the spring onions and potato and fry for 2 minutes. Add the thyme, squash and stock, bring to the boil, cover and simmer for 20 minutes.

2. Add the peas and chicken and cook for 5 minutes. Mash or blend to the desired consistency and stir in the Parmesan.

nutritional benefits of both
- *Nutritionally complete*
- *Provides vitamin A, vitamin C, iron (combination increases the absorption of iron), calcium and zinc*
- *Source of prebiotics*

country-style chicken & noodle soup

For that 'goodness in a bowl' craving, look no further than my special soup. I challenge any child not to feel comforted and content after this stand-out supper.

makes:
6 portions

1 tbsp olive oil
1 leek, chopped
40g red pepper, cut into 1cm dice
50g carrot, peeled and cut into
   1cm dice
50g butternut squash, peeled
   and cut into 1cm dice
1 tbsp plain flour

600ml homemade chicken stock
   (see page 142) or very low-salt
   chicken stock
25g baby (or fine egg) noodles
40g tiny broccoli florets
50g cooked chicken, cut into
   1.5cm pieces
2 tbsp double cream (*optional*)

1. Heat the oil in a pan. Add the leek, pepper, carrot and squash. Fry for 5 minutes. Add the flour, then blend in the stock. Bring up to the boil, then simmer for 10 minutes.

2. Meanwhile, cook the noodles according to the packet instructions, adding the broccoli florets 2 minutes before the end of the cooking time. Drain.

3. Add the chicken, noodles and broccoli to the vegetable and stock mixture, together with the cream, if using, and stir to combine.

nutritional benefits
- *Nutritionally complete*
- *Provides vitamin A, vitamin C, selenium and zinc*
- *Source of prebiotics*

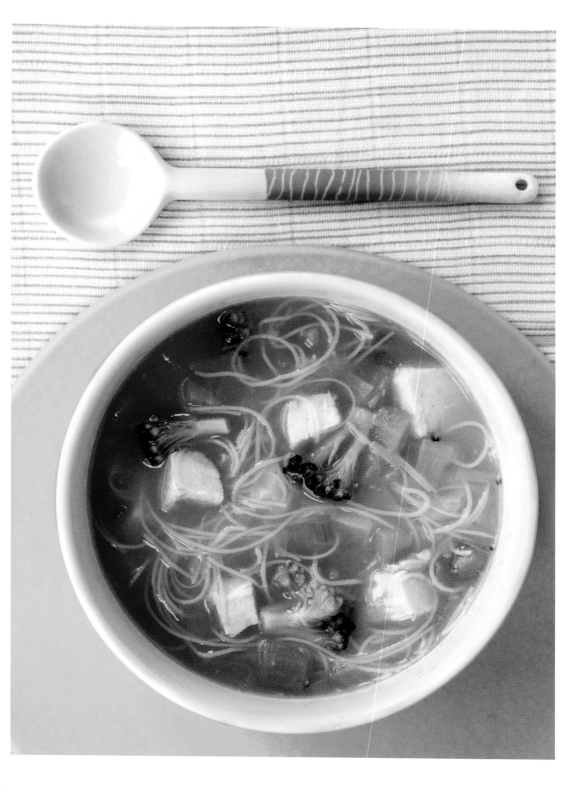

chicken stock

If you can, it's a good idea to make your own chicken stock, because unless you buy special very low-salt stock cubes, shop-bought versions often contain high levels of salt. This recipe is simple; just pop the ingredients into a pan and leave to simmer for around an hour. Then hey presto – fresh homemade stock!

makes:
approximately 1 litre

4 chicken thighs, boned and skinned
3 large carrots, peeled and sliced
2 leeks, sliced

1 large onion, sliced
1 celery stalk, sliced
2 sprigs fresh parsley
1 bouquet garni

1. Put all the ingredients into a large pan. Cover with 1 litre water. Bring to the boil, cover and simmer gently, for about 1 hour. Strain the stock through a sieve into a jug or bowl.

2. If you want to freeze, allow the strained stock to cool and pour into small containers. Transfer to the freezer.

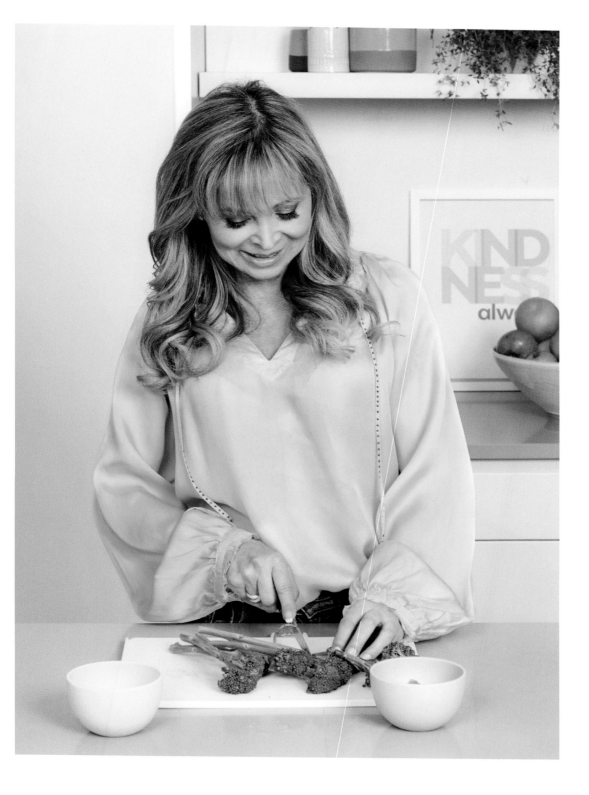

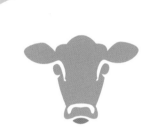

6–9 months
beef

beef with 5 veggies

The title says it all. This power packed dish contains not one but five veggies. And let's not sidestep the main ingredient here – iron-rich beef – which is a must on your tot's menu from 6 months.

makes:
4 portions

2 tsp sunflower oil
75g carrot, peeled and cut into 1cm dice
50g red pepper, peeled and cut into 1cm dice
100g leek, sliced

75g potatoes, peeled and cut into 1cm dice
125g minced beef
1 clove garlic, crushed
1 tbsp tomato purée
300ml very low-salt beef stock
25g spinach

1. Heat the oil in a pan. Add the carrot, pepper and leek and fry for 2 minutes.

2. Add the potatoes and mince and brown for 3–4 minutes.

3. Add the garlic and fry for 15 seconds. Add the tomato purée and stock, bring to a boil then cover and simmer for 20 minutes, until the meat and vegetables are cooked and tender

4. Add the spinach and stir until wilted. Blend to the desired consistency.

nutritional benefits
- *Nutritionally complete*
- *Provides vitamin A, vitamin C, iron (combination increases the absorption of iron), selenium and zinc*
- *Source of prebiotics*

beef & kale croquettes

Red meat is the best source of iron for your baby and there will no kicking up a fuss in getting this iron-rich dish gobbled up. These are also perfect for making ahead and freezing once cooked.

makes:
10 croquettes

25g kale
50g panko breadcrumbs
150g cold mashed potato (cooked without salt in the water)
2 spring onions, chopped
80g carrot, peeled and grated

25g Parmesan cheese, grated
1 tomato, deseeded and diced
75g cooked roast beef, diced
1 tsp chopped fresh thyme
1 egg, beaten
2 tbsp sunflower oil

1. Cook the kale in boiling water for 4 minutes. Drain and refresh under cold water. Dry and chop.

2. Place the cooked kale in a bowl with half the breadcrumbs, potato, spring onions, carrot, cheese, tomato, beef, thyme and egg. Mix together and shape into 10 croquettes. Roll in the remaining breadcrumbs.

3. Heat the oil in a frying pan. Fry the croquettes for 5–8 minutes until golden and heated through.

nutritional benefits
- *Nutritionally complete*
- *Provides vitamin A, vitamin C, iron (combination increases the absorption of iron), calcium, selenium and zinc*
- *Source of prebiotics*

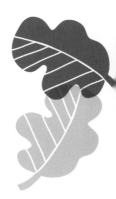

beef & kale purée

Iron is the critical nutrient required for the production of haemoglobin, which carries oxygen to your baby's developing brain and so it is easy to see why it's so essential. This is another recipe from my purée/finger food combo collection so with similar ingredients you can make croquettes, too (see opposite).

makes:
4 portions

150g minced beef
2 spring onions, sliced
80g carrot, peeled and diced
170g potatoes, peeled and diced

400g can chopped tomatoes
1 tsp chopped fresh thyme
25g kale, chopped
25g Parmesan cheese, grated

1. Put the minced beef into a pan. Heat the pan and brown the mince over a high heat, stirring. Add the spring onions, carrot and potatoes. Stir over the heat for 1–2 minutes.

2. Add the tomatoes, thyme and 150ml water. Bring to the boil, cover and simmer for 20 minutes.

3. Add the kale and simmer for 5 minutes. Stir in the Parmesan and blend or mash to the desired consistency.

nutritional benefits
- *Nutritionally complete*
- *Provides vitamin A, vitamin C, iron (combination increases the absorption of iron), calcium, selenium and zinc*
- *Source of prebiotics*

147

my first bolognese with 5 veggies

Spaghetti Bolognese will always be a children's favourite and I'm all for it! It's a fantastic quick, easy and nutritionally balanced family meal so let's get them started early.

makes:
3–4 portions

2 tsp sunflower oil
30g onion, finely diced
30g red pepper, cut into 1cm dice
30g carrot, peeled and cut into
  1cm dice
30g button mushrooms, cut into
  1cm dice
30g celery, cut into 1cm dice

100g lean minced beef
1 clove garlic, crushed
1 x 225g tin chopped tomatoes
100ml very low-salt beef stock
1 tsp tomato purée
mini pasta shells, to serve
  (*optional*)

1. Heat the oil in a pan. Add the diced vegetables and fry for 4–5 minutes. Add the mince and brown over the heat, stirring.

2. Add the garlic and fry for 10 seconds. Stir in the tomatoes, stock and tomato purée. Bring to the boil, cover and simmer for 30 minutes. Serve with mini pasta shells, if liked.

nutritional benefits
- *Good source of protein and together with pasta shells a Nutritionally complete*
- *Provides vitamin A, vitamin C, iron (combination increases the absorption of iron), selenium and zinc*
- *Source of prebiotics*

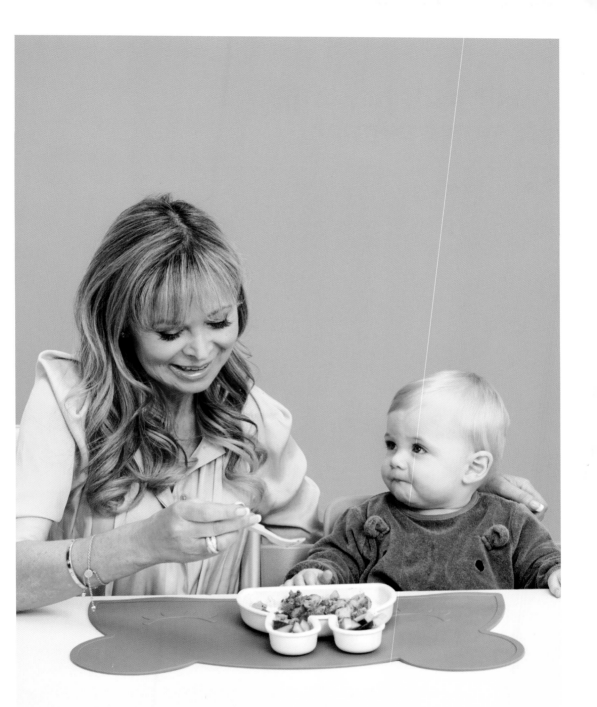

beef with parsnip & sweet pepper

Although red meat is a must, it can prove to be a slightly trickier texture for a baby to manage. By cooking slowly, the meat becomes soft and meltingly tender for her to eat. You could also save some of the beef, let it cool and serve as a nutritious finger food.

makes:
6 portions

1 tbsp sunflower oil
180g diced braising beef
1 onion, chopped
½ red pepper, cut into 1cm dice
1 tbsp plain flour

250ml very low-salt beef stock
1 parsnip, peeled and cut into 1cm dice
1 medium potato, peeled and cut into 1cm dice

1. Heat the oil in a pan. Add the beef and brown over a high heat. Transfer to a bowl. Add the onion and pepper and fry for 2 minutes, then stir through the flour and stock.

2. Return the beef to the pan with the diced parsnip and potato. Cover and simmer over a gentle heat for 1½ hours or until tender. Alternatively, transfer the beef to a casserole dish, cover and cook in an oven preheated to 150°C (fan 130°C/gas mark 2) for 1½ hours or until tender. Mash to the desired consistency.

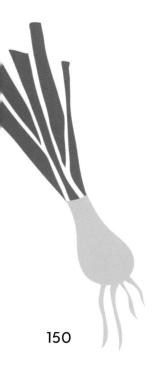

nutritional benefits
- *Nutritionally complete*
- *Good source of protein*
- *Provides vitamin A, vitamin C, iron (combination increases the absorption of iron) and zinc*
- *Source of prebiotics*

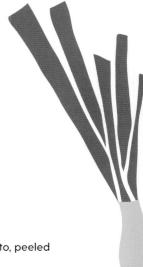

beef, carrot & sweet potato purée

Beef and veg flavoured with garlic make this dish a classic you will (I hope!) come back to again and again.

makes:
4 portions

1 tbsp sunflower oil
1 leek, chopped
100g carrots, peeled and diced
100g minced beef
1 clove garlic, crushed

100g sweet potato, peeled and diced
75g potato peeled and diced
1 tsp tomato purée
200ml very low-salt beef stock

1. Heat the oil in a pan. Add the leek and carrots and fry for 2 minutes, then add the beef. Fry until browned, stirring.

2. Add the garlic, sweet potato, potato and tomato purée. Gradually add the stock, stir, cover and simmer for 30 minutes. Mash or blend to the desired consistency.

nutritional benefits
- *Nutritionally complete*
- *Good source of protein*
- *Provides vitamin A, vitamin C, iron (combination increases the absorption of iron) and zinc*
- *Source of prebiotics*

mini meatballs with carrot & apple

These mini meatballs make the perfect finger food but you can also add them to a fresh tomato sauce and serve with spaghetti for a more complete meal for the rest of the family come dinner time. They are perfect served with the tomato sauce in the herby chicken goujons with tomato & basil sauce (see page 220). You can also freeze them once cooked.

makes:
30 balls

75g white bread or 50g panko breadcrumbs
1 onion, chopped
1 medium carrot, peeled and grated
1 eating apple, peeled and grated

1 tsp chopped fresh thyme
1 clove garlic, crushed
40g Parmesan cheese, grated
225g lean minced beef
sunflower oil, for frying

1. Whiz the white bread in a food processor until you have fine crumbs or place the dried breadcrumbs in the processor. Add the onion, carrot and apple, thyme, garlic, Parmesan and minced beef. Whiz for a few seconds until just combined.

2. Using your hands, shape the mixture into thirty meatballs. Heat a little oil in a large non-stick frying pan and fry the balls, in batches, for 4–5 minutes on each side until golden and cooked through. Alternatively you could cook the balls on a lightly oiled tray in a 200°C (fan 180 °C/gas mark 6) oven for 15–20 minutes or until cooked, turning halfway through.

nutritional benefits
- *Good source of protein*
- *Provides vitamin A, vitamin C, iron (combination increases the absorption of iron) and zinc*
- *Source of prebiotics*

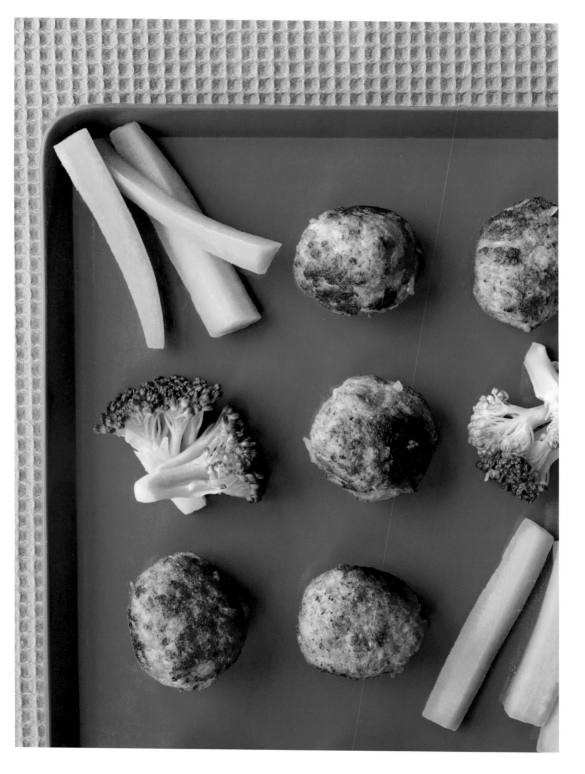

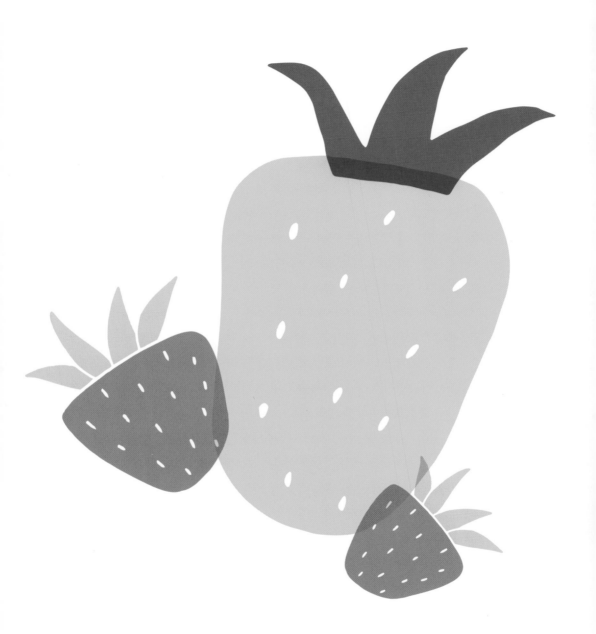

chapter 4

recipes for growing independence

9–12 MONTHS

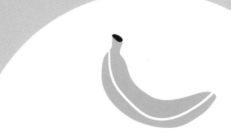

9–12 months
breakfast

baby muesli

This baby-friendly brekkie will soon be a morning staple –
not only can you make a big batch and store in a jar until
you need but it's incredibly nourishing for your little one.

makes:
3–4 portions

50g porridge oats
1 tsp chia seeds
1 tsp flax seeds
1 tsp pumpkin seeds
15g raisins

30g soft dried apple, chopped into
   tiny pieces
a pinch of ground cinnamon
milk, to serve

1. Place all of the ingredients in a lidded jar or airtight container.
    Put the lid on, shake well and store until needed.

2. Spoon the muesli into a bowl, add the milk and stir.

nutritional benefits
*   *Provides vitamin C, iron (combination increases the
    absorption of iron), omega 3s, zinc, manganese*
*   *Source of prebiotics*

157

yoghurt pancakes with berries

These pancakes will tempt even the fussiest eaters to chomp away their breakfast. Plus, you'll be happy too as these pancakes (pictured on pp160–1) are free from refined sugar and provide a host of nutrients.

makes:
about 30
mini pancakes

1 egg, beaten
350g Greek yoghurt
150ml milk
200g self-raising flour
1 overripe banana, mashed

sunflower oil, for frying
a knob of unsalted butter
raspberries and blueberries,
   to serve

1. Place the egg, yoghurt and milk in a bowl and stir to combine. Add the flour and banana and whisk until smooth.

2. Heat a little oil in a large non-stick frying pan. Add the butter and when it is foaming, add large heaped tablespoons of the mixture to the pan. Cook for 2 minutes, then flip over and cook for another 1–2 minutes until golden brown and cooked through. (You should be able to get 5–6 pancakes in the pan at one go, so cook in batches.)

3. Serve with raspberries and blueberries.

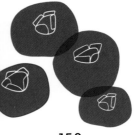

nutritional benefits
- *Nutritionally complete*
- *Provides vitamin D, vitamin C, iron (combination increases the absorption of iron) and calcium*

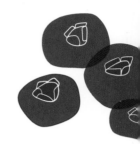

banana, blueberry & coconut pancakes

Who doesn't love pancakes? Whilst commonly seen as a 'treat' food, I've turned this into a power-packed breakfast for babies. Super fuel at its best!

makes:
6–8 pancakes

1 ripe banana
1 egg
50g porridge oats
20g desiccated coconut
a few drops of pure vanilla extract

100ml milk
75g blueberries
sunflower oil, for frying
a knob of unsalted butter, for frying

1. Place all the ingredients, except the blueberries, into a jug. Blend until smooth using an electric stick blender. Add the blueberries.

2. Heat a little oil in a large non-stick frying pan. Add the butter and when it is foaming, add large heaped tablespoons of the mixture to the pan. Cook for 2 minutes, then flip over and cook for another 1–2 minutes until golden brown and cooked through. (You should be able to get 5–6 pancakes in the pan at one go, so cook in batches.)

nutritional benefits
- *Nutritionally complete*
- *Provides vitamin A, vitamin C, calcium and iodine*
- *Source of prebiotics*

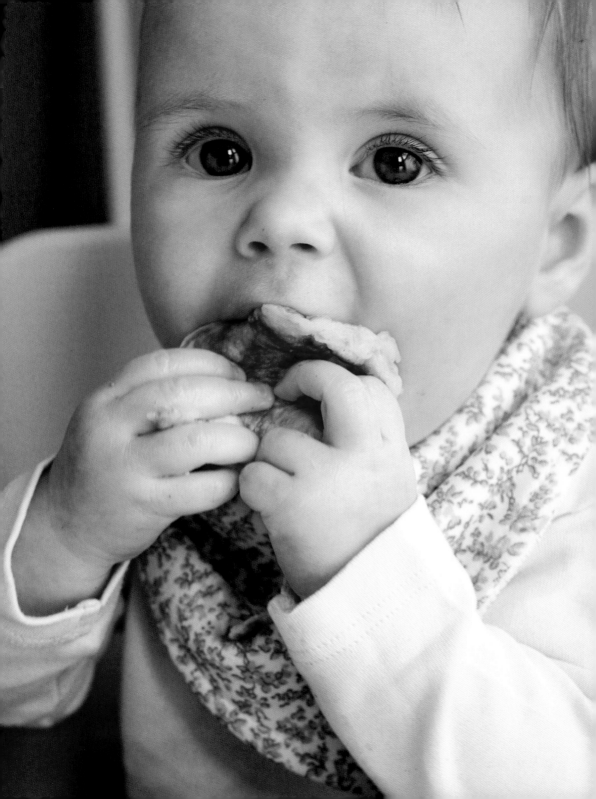

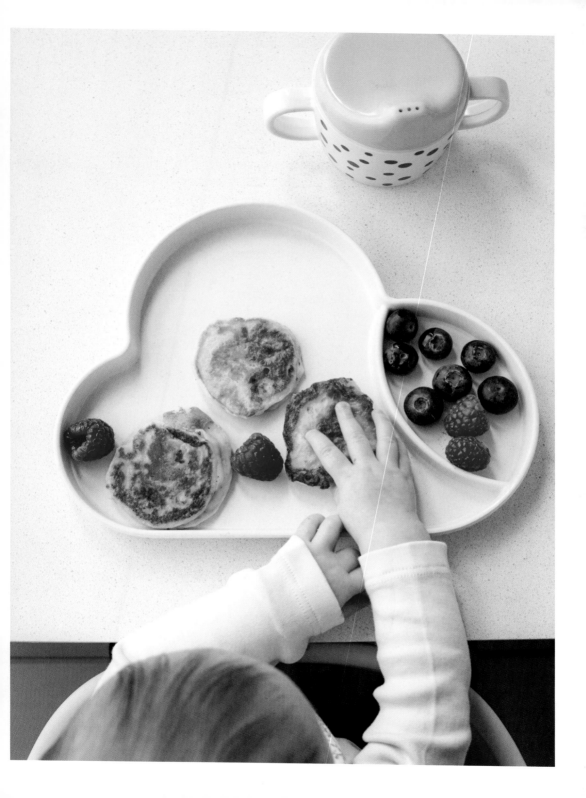

yoghurt, banana & seed loaf

This lovely loaf is a great alternative to toast – packed full of grated carrots, raisins and seeds it makes a tasty breakfast or mid-morning snack. So tasty, in fact, that you'll want to pack it in your own lunchbox too.

makes:
8 slices

You will also need:
900g loaf tin

75g unsalted butter, at room temperature, plus extra for greasing
50g caster sugar
2 eggs
100g self-raising flour
40g ground almonds
1 tsp baking powder
75g natural yoghurt
1 small banana, mashed
100g carrot, peeled and grated
100g raisins
1 tbsp flax seeds
2 tbsp pumpkin seeds

1. Preheat the oven to 180°C (fan 160°C/gas mark 4). Grease and line the loaf tin with baking parchment.

2. Put all the ingredients, except the raisins and seeds, into a bowl. Whisk until light and fluffy. Stir in the raisins. Spoon into the tin. Sprinkle with seeds.

3. Bake for 55 minutes until well risen and light golden. Insert a skewer into the centre to make sure it is cooked – it should come out clean.

4. Leave to cool in the tin for 5 minutes, then turn out and allow to cool on a wire rack before cutting into slices.

nutritional benefits
- *Nutritionally complete*
- *Provides vitamin E, B vitamins, vitamin A, calcium and omega 3s, zinc and selenium*
- *Source of prebiotics*

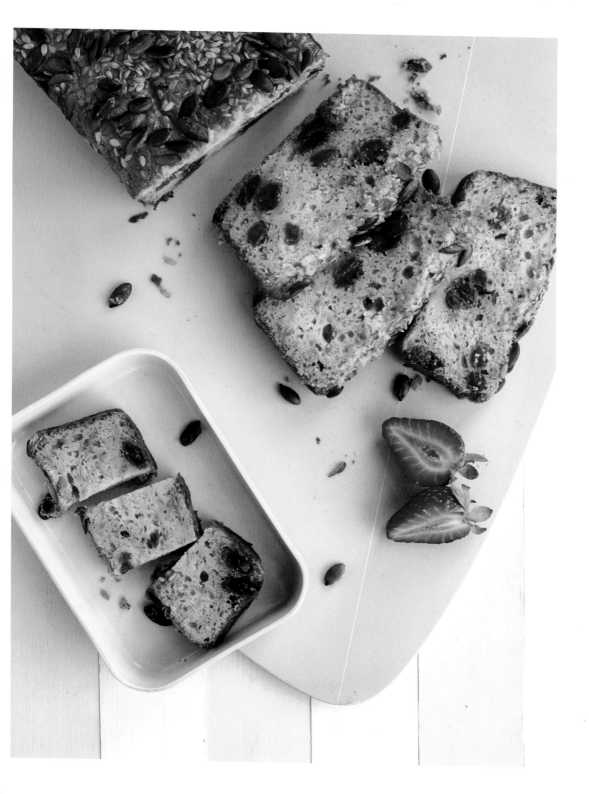

soft boiled egg with welsh rarebit toast

Now that runny eggs are deemed safe for babies to eat (make sure to look out for the British Lion stamp, see page 45), dippy eggs are back on the menu! I like to serve it with Welsh rarebit or you can simply make soldiers out of toast.

makes:
1 adult and
1 baby portion

15g unsalted butter
1 tbsp plain flour
80ml milk
1 egg yolk

25g Parmesan cheese, grated
1 tsp chopped fresh chives
2 slices of bread
2 eggs

1. Preheat the grill to high.

2. Melt the butter in a small pan. Add the flour and stir over the heat for a few seconds. Add the milk, whisking until smooth and thickened. Add the cheese and stir until melted. Remove from the heat and stir in the egg yolk and chives.

3. Lightly toast the bread until golden. Spread the cheese mixture over both slices of toast. Place on a baking tray. Place under the grill for 5–8 minutes until bubbling and golden. Cut into triangles.

4. Put the eggs into a pan of cold water. Bring up to the boil. Boil rapidly for 4–5 minutes. Place in egg cups and slice off the top. Serve with the Welsh rarebit.

nutritional benefits
- *Provides, vitamin D, vitamin E, calcium, iron*
- *Source of prebiotics*

banana eggy bread

Banana eggy bread? Confused? Don't be. It really does work and I promise your baby will love this super-charged brekkie.

makes:
12 fingers

1 small ripe banana, mashed
1 tbsp milk
1 egg, beaten

4 slices of raisin or fruit bread
sunflower oil, for frying
a knob of unsalted butter

1. Mix the banana, milk and egg together in a bowl. Cut each slice of bread into three fingers. Dip the fingers quickly into the banana mixture.

2. Heat the oil in a large non-stick frying pan. Add the butter and when it is foaming, add the bread. Fry for 1–2 minutes on each side until golden and cooked through. (You will need to cook in two batches.)

nutritional benefits

- *Nutritionally complete*

- *Provides, vitamin D, vitamin E, vitamin B6, potassium, magnesium and iron*

overnight oats with berries & seeds

This only needs a few minutes of prep the night before – simply stir everything together and then leave in the fridge for this recipe to work its magic.

makes:
1 portion

30g porridge oats
3 tbsp apple juice
3 tbsp milk
1 tsp chia seeds
1 tsp pumpkin seeds

maple syrup, to taste
25g raspberries
25g blueberries,
    chopped (see page 46)

1. Place the oats, juice, milk and seeds in a bowl. Cover and leave in the fridge overnight.

2. In the morning, stir together adding a little maple syrup, to taste. Serve with fresh berries.

nutritional benefits
- *Nutritionally complete*
- *Provides omega 3s, zinc, calcium and vitamin C, some iron (combination increases the absorption of iron)*
- *Source of prebiotics*

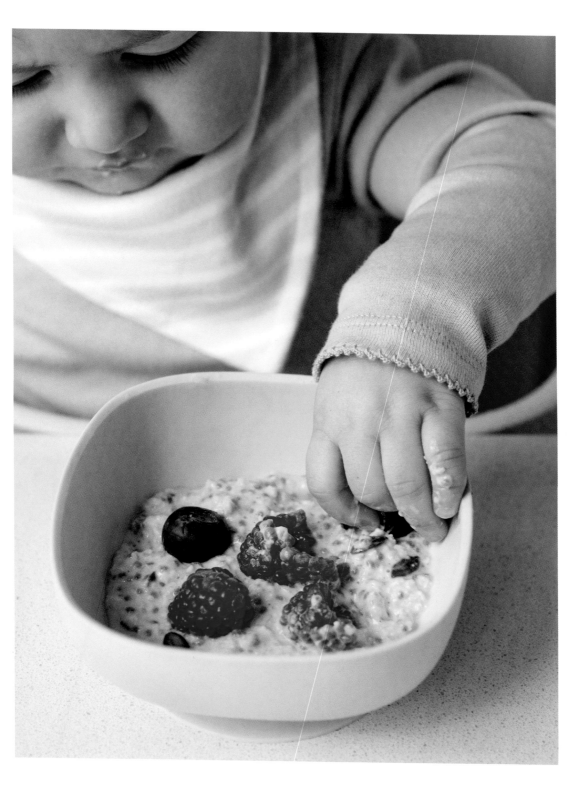

squash, banana & pumpkin seed muffins

Mini muffins are my go-to whether it's for breakfast, lunch or snacks for when I'm in the office or on the go. And these are one of my favourites. These mini marvels can be frozen and contain so much goodness including vitamin E, B vitamins, vitamin A, calcium, omega 3s, selenium and zinc so if your baby is going through a difficult eating stage this recipe is one for you.

makes:
24 mini muffins

....

You will also need
24 hole mini muffin tin

24 paper mini muffin cases

75g unsalted butter, at room temperature
50g light brown sugar
2 eggs
125g self-raising flour
1 tsp baking powder

75g natural yoghurt
1 ripe banana, mashed
100g butternut squash, peeled and grated
1 tsp mixed spice
25g pumpkin seeds

1. Preheat the oven to 180°C (fan 160°C/gas mark 4). Line the muffin tin with the paper cases.

2. Place all the ingredients, except the pumpkin seeds, into a bowl. Whisk until with an electric hand-held whisk, until well combined. Spoon the mixture into the paper cases. Sprinkle with seeds.

3. Bake in the oven for 15–20 minutes or until well risen and light golden. Allow to cool on a wire rack. These can be stored for up to 3 days in an airtight container.

nutritional benefits
- *Nutritionally complete*
- *Provides vitamin E, B vitamins, vitamin A, calcium and omega 3s, selenium and zinc*
- *Source of prebiotics*

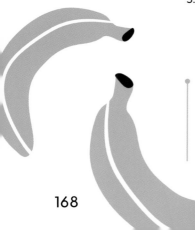

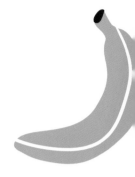

banana & oat waffles

All hail the waffle! These are made using bananas instead of sugar, for sweetness, and porridge oats replace flour. You'll need a waffle maker for these but it will be a family pleaser for years to come. Plus, you'll also be able to make my favourite sweet potato & carrot waffles (see page 186).

makes:
4 waffles

225g ripe bananas, mashed
80g porridge oats
2 large eggs
1 tsp pure vanilla extract

1 tsp baking powder
sunflower oil, for greasing
sliced banana and berries,
  to serve

1. Preheat a waffle maker.

2. Place all the ingredients in a bowl. Whisk until smooth.

3. Brush the waffle maker plate with a little oil.

4. Spoon a quarter of the mixture into the centre of the plate, spread it out, pushing to the edges.

5. Close the waffle maker lid and leave for 5 minutes before lifting. The waffle should be golden and cooked through. Repeat to make four waffles in total. Serve with sliced banana and berries.

nutritional benefits
- *Nutritionally complete*
- *Provides vitamin B6, vitamin C and iron (combination increases the absorption of iron)*
- *Source of prebiotics*

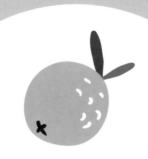

9–12 months
fruit

berry fool

You would be a fool not to try this fruity number!
Fresh and zingy with lots of blueberries, raspberries
and blackberries which are paired with creamy
Greek yoghurt – it's simply delicious.

makes:
4 portions

150g blueberries
100g raspberries
50g blackberries
1 tsp maple syrup, plus extra
   to taste

3 tbsp mascarpone cream
200g Greek natural yoghurt
1 tsp pure vanilla extract

1. Put the berries into a pan with 1 tsp of maple syrup. Heat for a
   few minutes until the berries have burst. Stir until softened, then
   pour into sieve placed over a bowl and press the fruit through
   the sieve with a spoon. Leave to cool.

2. Stir the mascarpone in a bowl with the yoghurt and vanilla
   and maple syrup, to taste.

3. Stir in the cold fruit purée, pour into four dishes and chill for
   2 hours.

nutritional benefits
- *Contains vitamin C, vitamin B, calcium and iodine*
- *Source of prebiotics*

apple & berry crumble

Who doesn't love a classic crumble? This one is bursting
with a gooey apple and berry filling. It's full of antioxidants
from the berries and fibre from the apple as well as
vitamin C and B vitamins, too.

makes:
6 portions

a knob of unsalted butter
2 sweet eating apples, eg
   Pink Lady or Braeburn, peeled
   and cut into 1.5cm dice
1 tbsp maple syrup
15g brown sugar
150g raspberries
100g blueberries
100g blackberries

FOR THE TOPPING
75g plain flour
20g porridge oats
50g unsalted butter, diced
15g brown sugar
1 tsp chia seeds

1. Preheat the oven to 200°C (fan 180°C/gas mark 6).

2. Heat the butter in a pan and add the diced apple, maple syrup
   and sugar. Cook for 8 minutes, stirring. Remove from the heat
   and stir in the berries. Spoon the fruit mixture into one large
   ovenproof dish or six small ovenproof dishes.

3. Place the topping ingredients into a bowl. Rub the butter into
   the dry ingredients using your fingers. Sprinkle the topping over
   the fruit.

4. Bake for 20 minutes in the oven until bubbling and the fruits
   are soft.

nutritional benefits
- *Provides vitamin C and B vitamins*
- *Source of prebiotics*

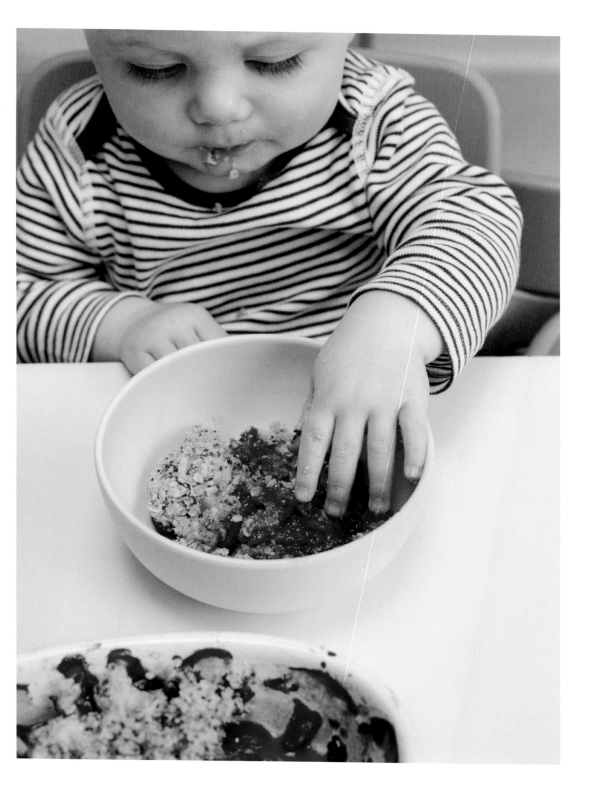

fruity lollies

Bursting with vitamins and minerals these fresh and fruity lollies are great for teething and a fantastic way to make sure your baby is getting lots of essential nutrients in their diet.

And, if you offer any of these vitamin-C rich lollies after your baby has eaten a meal containing non-haem iron (a vegetarian source of iron), it can help to increase iron absorption. Lollies all round! Pictured on pages 176–7.

beetroot, strawberry & blueberry lollies

makes:
6 ice lollies

You will also need
6 ice lolly moulds

50g cooked beetroot, diced
80g strawberries, chopped

100g blueberries, chopped
100ml apple juice

1. Place all the ingredients in a jug. Blend using an electric stick blender until smooth.

2. Pour into six ice lolly moulds and freeze for 5 hours.

nutritional benefits
• *Provides vitamins A and C and B vitamins*

carrot, mango & orange lollies

makes:
6 ice lollies

You will also need
6 ice lolly moulds

50g carrot, peeled and chopped
150g mango, peeled and
    chopped

1 orange, peeled, skin and pith
    removed and diced
100ml apple juice

1. Place all the ingredients in a food processor or blender. Blend until smooth and runny.

2. Pour into six ice lolly moulds and freeze for 5 hours.

nutritional benefits
- *Provides vitamins A and C*

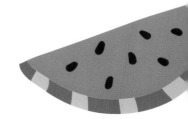

watermelon & kiwi layer lollies

makes:
6 ice lollies

You will also need
6 ice lolly moulds

300g ripe watermelon, peeled,
    deseeded and diced

3 ripe kiwi fruit, peeled, cored
    and diced

1. Put the watermelon cubes into a food processor. Whiz until completely smooth and runny. Divide between six ice lolly moulds, filling up to three quarters of each mould. Freeze for 2 hours.

2. Put the diced kiwi fruit into the food processor. Whiz until smooth. Pour into six ice lolly moulds, filling to the top of each mould. Freeze for 4 hours or until completely frozen.

nutritional benefits
- *Provides vitamins A and C*

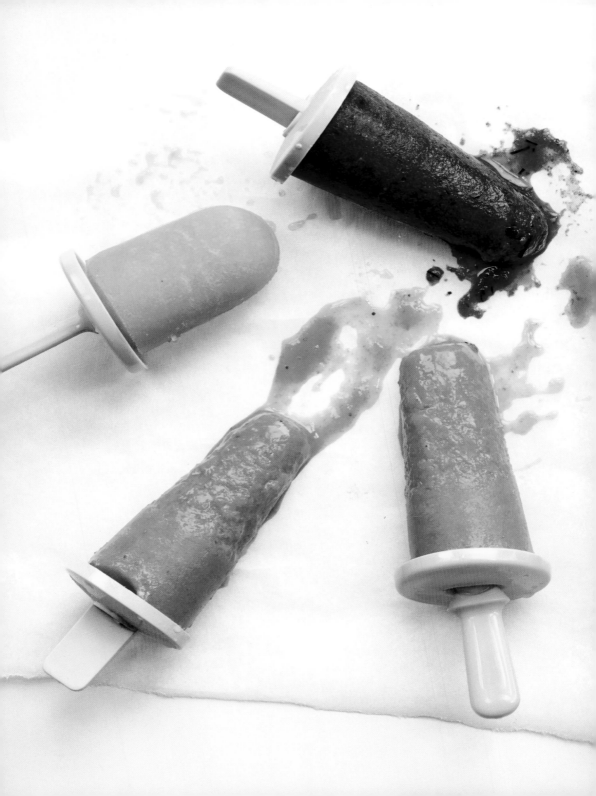

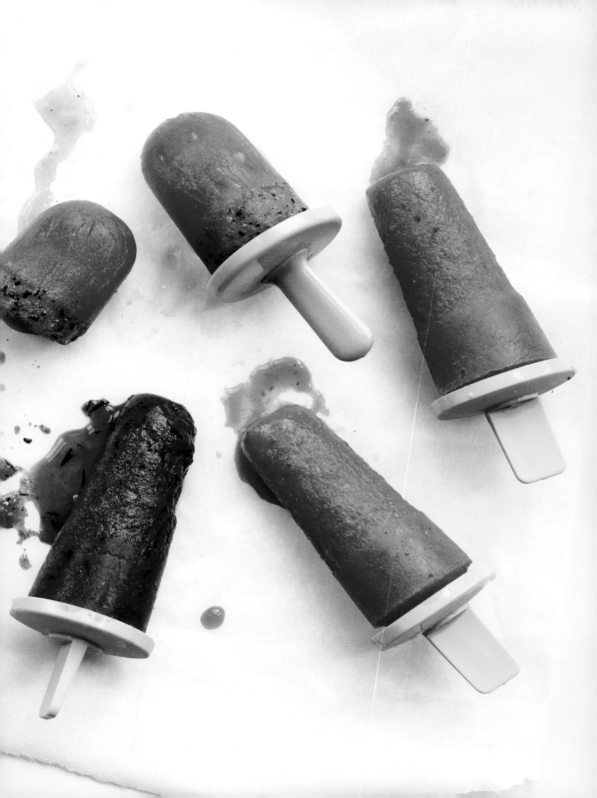

mango, strawberry & melon lollies

makes:
2 ice lollies

You will also need
2 ice lolly moulds

50g ripe mango, peeled and diced
30g strawberries, diced

50g cantaloupe melon, peeled and diced

1. Put the mango into a small processor and blend until puréed and completely smooth, then pour into a bowl.

2. Add the strawberries and melon. Mix together and pour into two lolly moulds. Freeze for 6 hours or until completely frozen.

nutritional benefits
- *Provides vitamins A and C and B vitamins*

mango, papaya, banana & strawberry lollies

makes:
4 ice lollies

You will also need
4 ice lolly moulds

150g mixed mango and papaya, peeled and diced

100g ripe banana, sliced
50g strawberries, sliced

1. Place all the ingredients in a jug. Blend using an electric stick blender until smooth.

2. Pour into four lolly moulds and freeze for 6 hours.

nutritional benefits
- *Provides vitamin A, vitamin C, vitamin B6*

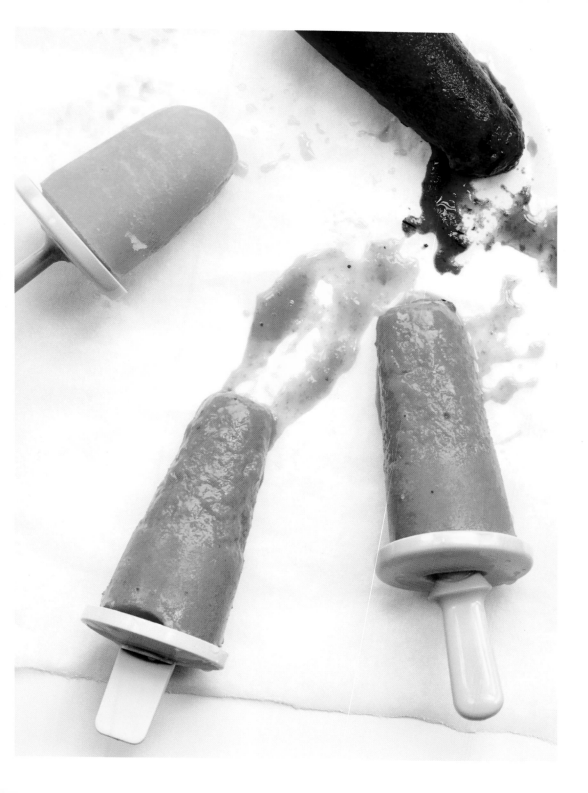

9–12 months
vegetables

bulgur wheat with tomato & lentil sauce

Bulgur wheat is a good source of carbohydrate for your growing baby, and it's another new texture to explore.

makes:
4 portions

50g bulgur wheat
1 tsp sunflower oil
½ red onion, chopped
40g red lentils
2 tomatoes, cut into 1cm dice

2 tsp tomato purée
200ml homemade vegetable stock (see page 105), very low-salt vegetable stock or water
15g Parmesan cheese, grated

1. Put the bulgur wheat into a small pan with 100ml of water. Cover and bring up to the boil. Turn off the heat and set aside for 20 minutes or until the water is absorbed.

2. Meanwhile, heat the oil in a pan. Add the onion and fry for 2 minutes. Add the lentils and tomatoes and toss in the heat for 30 seconds. Add the tomato purée and stock. Cover and simmer for 15 minutes. Blend until smooth. Stir in the Parmesan.

3. Mix the bulgur wheat with the sauce.

nutritional benefits
- *Nutritionally complete*
- *Provides vitamin C, iron (combination increases the absorption of iron) and zinc*
- *Source of prebiotics*

broccoli, sweet potato & chickpea croquettes

Chickpeas are a good source of protein and iron, so batch cook these for a quick and nutritious lunch or snack. You can also freeze them once cooked.

makes:
15 croquettes

1 x 250g sweet potato
75g small broccoli florets
75g tinned chickpeas
50g carrots, peeled and grated
25g Parmesan cheese, grated

4 spring onions, chopped
1 egg yolk
60g panko breadcrumbs
sunflower oil, for drizzling

1. Preheat the oven to 180°C (fan 160°C/gas mark 4). Line a baking tray with baking parchment.

2. Scrub and prick the potato with a sharp knife. Cook the whole potato in the microwave for 8 minutes or until soft. Alternatively preheat the oven to 200°C (fan 180°C/gas mark 6), and roast the sweet potato in the oven for 50 minutes until tender. Leave to cool, then scoop out the flesh. Steam the broccoli for 4 minutes.

4. Place the sweet potato flesh, broccoli, chickpeas, carrots, cheese, spring onions, egg yolk and 30g of the breadcrumbs in a food processor. Whiz until roughly chopped. Shape into fifteen croquettes. Roll each croquette in the remaining breadcrumbs.

5. Place on the baking tray. Drizzle with oil and bake for 15 minutes. Turn over and bake for another 10 minutes until lightly golden.

nutritional benefits
- *Nutritionally complete*
- *Provides vitamin A, calcium, vitamin C, iron (combination increases the absorption of iron) and zinc*
- *Source of prebiotics*

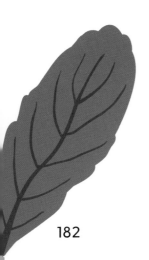

chickpea pancakes

These pancakes are bursting with nutrients and are super tasty too. They also freeze well once cooked so make the full batch and save some for the weekend as the whole family can (and will!) gobble these up.

makes:
10–12 pancakes

100g tinned chickpeas
40g carrot, peeled and grated
30g baby spinach, roughly
  chopped
2 eggs

100g self-raising flour
150ml milk
1–2 tbsp sweet chilli sauce
40g Parmesan cheese, grated
sunflower oil, for frying

1. Put the chickpeas into a food processor. Whiz for a few seconds until roughly chopped. Add the remaining ingredients. Whiz for 5 seconds until finely chopped and blended.

2. Heat a little sunflower oil in a large non-stick frying pan. Add large tablespoons of mixture to the pan. Fry for 2–3 minutes, on each side, until golden and cooked through. (You will need to do this in batches.)

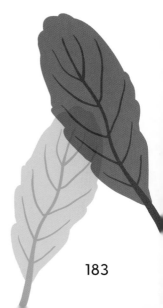

nutritional benefits
- *Nutritionally complete*
- *Provides vitamin A, calcium, iron and zinc*
- *Source of prebiotics*

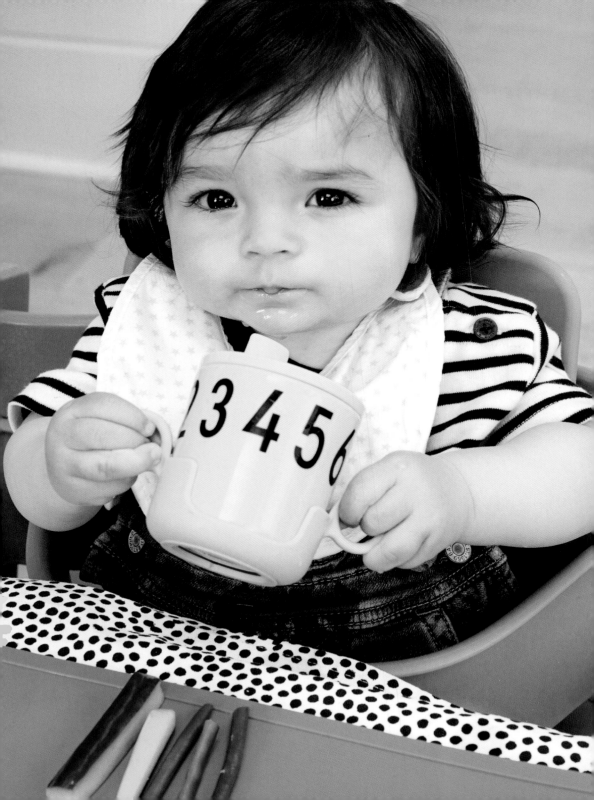

lentil, sweet potato & kale with tomatoes

Lentils are a good source of iron for your baby but you do need to pair any vegetarian iron sources with vitamin C as this lends a helping hand to your baby's body in absorbing iron. The chopped tomatoes and kale will do just the job here.

makes:
4 portions

2 tsp sunflower oil
1 red onion, chopped
1 large sweet potato, peeled and cut into 1.5cm dice
50g red lentils

400g tin chopped tomatoes
250ml homemade vegetable stock (see page 105), very low-salt vegetable stock or water
30g kale

1. Heat the oil in a pan. Add the red onion and fry for 3 minutes. Add the diced potato, lentils, tomatoes and stock. Cover and simmer for 15 minutes.

2. Add the kale, cover and simmer for another 8 minutes, until tender. Blend or mash to the desired consistency.

nutritional benefits
- *Nutritionally complete*
- *Provides vitamin A, vitamin C, iron (combination increases the absorption of iron) calcium and zinc*
- *Source of prebiotics*

185

sweet potato & carrot waffles

I've given this traditional sweet treat a nutritious makeover by using grated carrot and sweet potato, but little ones will still lap them up! You will need a waffle maker for these, but you'll also be able to make my banana & oat waffles recipe (see page 169).

makes:
6 waffles

125g carrots, peeled and grated
175g sweet potato, peeled and grated
100g Parmesan cheese, grated
3 spring onions, finely chopped
1 tsp chopped fresh thyme
3 eggs, beaten
70g self-raising flour
sunflower oil, for greasing

1. Preheat a waffle maker.

2. Put all the ingredients into a mixing bowl and stir well, to combine.

3. Brush the waffle maker with sunflower oil. Put one-sixth of the mixture into the centre of the waffle plate. Spread out a little, pushing the mixture to the edges.

4. Close the lid and leave for 5 minutes before lifting. The waffle should be golden and cooked through. Repeat to make six waffles in total.

nutritional benefits
- *Provides vitamin A, vitamin E, calcium and iron*
- *Source of prebiotics*

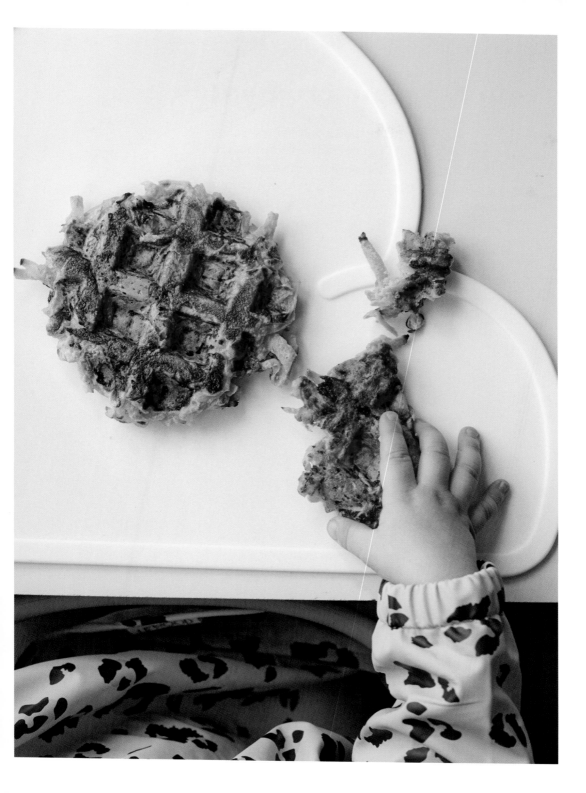

tofu & veggie croquettes

Tofu is a high protein superfood containing calcium,
iron and zinc which are critical nutrients for all babies.
And when combined with veggies, panko breadcrumbs
and a sprinkling of basil, you get a delicious croquette.
Finger food at its best! You can also freeze them
once cooked.

makes:
10 croquettes

150g cold mashed potato (cooked
   without salt in the water)
2 spring onions, sliced
25g Parmesan cheese, grated
50g panko breadcrumbs
75g firm tofu, grated

50g carrot, peeled and grated
75g brown mushrooms, roughly
   chopped
1 tbsp chopped fresh basil
1 egg, beaten
2 tbsp sunflower oil

1. Place the potato, spring onions, cheese, half the breadcrumbs,
   tofu, carrot, mushrooms, basil and egg in a bowl. Stir thoroughly
   to combine and shape into ten croquettes. Roll in the remaining
   breadcrumbs.

2. Heat the oil in a large non-stick frying pan. Fry the croquettes for
   5–8 minutes until golden and heated through.

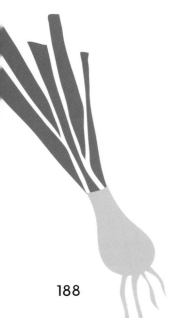

nutritional benefits
- *Nutritionally complete*
- *Provides vitamin A, vitamin C, calcium, iron and zinc*
- *Source of prebiotics*

parsnip, squash & chia fritters

This recipe is quick, easy and nutritious. Simply add your grated root veggies to the bowl with chia seeds, curry powder and beaten eggs, et voilà – quick as a flash fritters for hungry baby.

makes:
18 fritters

3 eggs, beaten
150g parsnips, peeled and grated
150g butternut squash, peeled and grated

1 tbsp chia seeds
a good pinch of curry powder
sunflower oil, for frying

1. Put the eggs into a large mixing bowl. Add the grated vegetables, chia seeds and curry powder. Mix well.

2. Heat a little oil in a large non-stick frying pan. Add small spoonfuls of the mixture to the pan and fry for 2–3 minutes and then flip over and fry for another 2–3 minutes until cooked through. (This is best done in batches.)

nutritional benefits
· *Good source of protein*
· *Provides omega 3s, vitamins A and C and iron*

frittata muffins

A frittata in the shape of a muffin you say? Yes!
These protein-packed little gems are super simple to
make and much easier for little hands to manage than
a traditional slice.

makes:
12 muffins

....

You will also need
12 hole non-stick or
silicone muffin tin

sunflower oil, for greasing
100g new potatoes
5 large eggs
75g Cheddar cheese, grated

4 spring onions, chopped
50g frozen peas
6 cherry tomatoes, chopped

1. Preheat the oven to 200°C (fan 180°C/gas mark 6). Grease a 12-hole muffin tin with oil.

2. Cook the new potatoes in boiling water for 12–15 minutes. Drain, cool and cut into 1cm dice.

3. Beat the eggs in a large bowl. Stir in the diced potatoes, cheese, spring onions, peas and tomatoes. Pour the mixture into the muffin tin moulds.

4. Bake for 20–25 minutes until well risen and golden. Leave to cool for 5 minutes in the tin, then release from the tin and cool on a wire rack.

nutritional benefits
- *Nutritionally complete*
- *Provides vitamin D, vitamin E, vitamin C, iron (combination increases the absorption of iron), calcium, iodine*
- *Source of prebiotics*

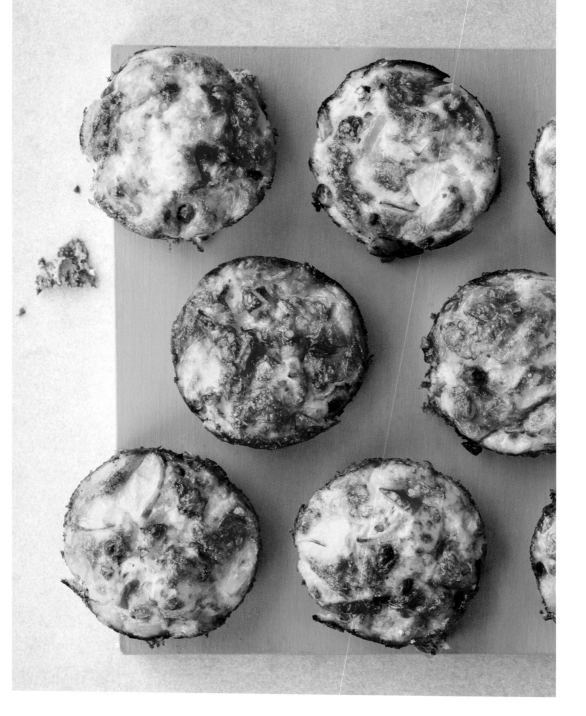

brown rice, squash, lentil & tomato

Brown rice and lentils are good sources of the antioxidant selenium which plays an important role in supporting your baby's immune system. This dish also boasts vitamin A, vitamin C, calcium, iron and zinc to help give your growing baby the very best start.

makes:
4 portions

50g brown rice
a knob of unsalted butter
1 onion, chopped
100g butternut squash, peeled
  and diced

1 clove garlic, crushed
2 tomatoes, skinned and diced
50g cooked Puy lentils
1 tbsp chopped fresh basil
1 tbsp grated Parmesan cheese

1. Cook the rice according to the packet instructions. Drain.

2. Heat the butter in a non-stick frying pan. Add the onion and squash and fry for 5 minutes.

3. Add the garlic to the frying pan and cook for 10 seconds. Add the tomatoes and stir until soft. Add the cooked rice, lentils, basil and cheese. Stir until well mixed.

nutritional benefits
- *Nutritionally complete*
- *Provides vitamin A, vitamin C, iron (combination increases the absorption of iron), calcium and zinc*
- *Source of prebiotics*

roasted vegetables with baby shell pasta

Don't delay introducing texture. And why would you when you can give your baby super-yummy recipes like this? Roasting the veggies gives them a delicious natural sweetness, and when combined with baby pasta shells, it's the perfect way to try new textures.

makes:
4 portions

75g red pepper, cut into 1.5cm dice
75g small cauliflower florets
75g squash, peeled and cut into 1.5cm dice
75g courgette, diced

2 tsp olive oil
75g baby pasta shells
2 tbsp cream cheese
25g Parmesan cheese, grated

1. Preheat the oven to 220°C (fan 200°C/gas mark 7). Line a baking tray with baking parchment.

2. Put the vegetables on the lined tray and drizzle the oil over. Roast in the oven for 20 minutes.

3. Cook the pasta according to the packet instructions. Drain, reserving 3 tablespoons of the cooking water.

4. Tip the pasta back into the pan with the roasted vegetables, cream cheese, Parmesan and reserved cooking water. Stir until the pasta is coated in the sauce.

nutritional benefits
- *Nutritionally complete*
- *Provides vitamin A, folic acid, vitamin C, calcium and iodine*
- *Source of prebiotics*

cauliflower couscous, kale & lentils

It's important to start your baby on bitter savoury flavours from 6 months onwards, and this power-packed veggie medley is a great recipe to continue banging the drum for those bona fide superfoods!

makes:
4 portions

50g small broccoli florets
20g kale
200g small cauliflower florets
1 tbsp oil

a knob of unsalted butter
30g cooked Puy lentils
1 clove garlic, crushed

1. Steam the broccoli florets for 4 minutes.

2. Put the kale and cauliflower in a food processor. Whiz until finely chopped.

3. Heat the oil and butter in a large non-stick frying pan. Add the garlic and fry for 10 seconds before adding the kale and cauliflower. Fry for 5 minutes, until soft. Add the Puy lentils and broccoli, stir until heated through.

nutritional benefits
- *Nutritionally complete*
- *Provides vitamin A, folic acid, vitamin C, iron (combination increases the absorption of iron) and zinc*
- *Source of prebiotics*

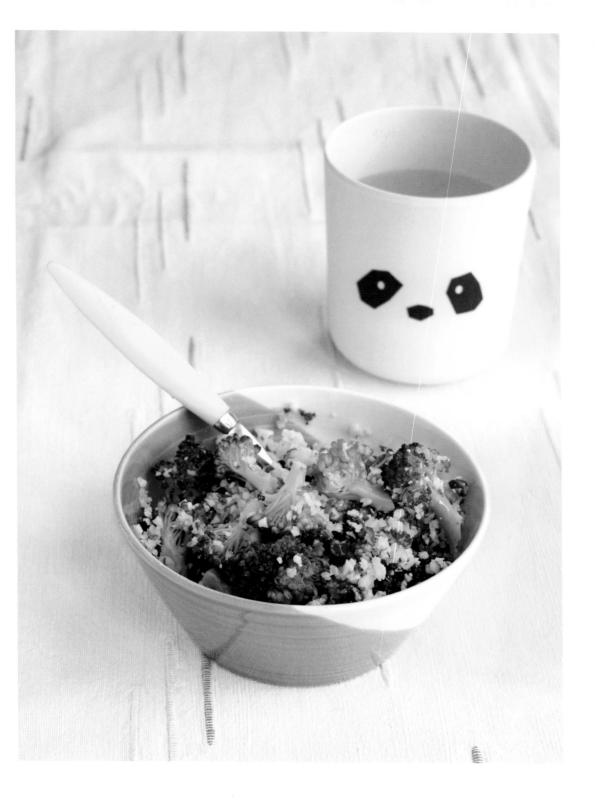

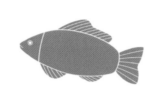

9-12 months
fish

scrummy salmon noodles with veggies

Food needs to look good before little ones will go in for the win, so why not serve up this scrummy salmon dish complete with a funny face using the baby corn, red pepper and peas.

makes:
2–3 portions

1 x 50g nest of egg noodles
20g frozen peas
2 tsp sunflower oil
¼ onion, sliced
½ small red pepper, cut into
  1cm dice
4 baby corn, sliced into rounds

½ clove garlic, crushed
100g salmon fillet, skinned, all
  bones removed and cut into
  1.5cm dice
1½ tbsp apple juice
1 tsp reduced salt soy sauce
a squeeze of lemon juice

1. Cook the noodles according to the packet instructions, stirring in the peas in the last 3 minutes of cooking time. Drain.

2. Heat the oil in a small frying pan. Add the onion, pepper and corn. Fry for 3–4 minutes. Add the garlic and salmon. Cook for 5 minutes until cooked through.

3. Add the cooked peas, cooked noodles, apple juice, soy sauce and lemon juice. Toss together over the heat.

nutritional benefits

- *Nutritionally complete*
- *Provides vitamin A, vitamin C, iron (combination increases the absorption of iron), omega 3s, iodine and zinc*
- *Source of prebiotics*

tuna, butternut squash & sweetcorn croquettes

Easy to pick up with a soft texture and crispy coating, my croquettes are perfect for babies and are sure to be a hit with older children too. You can make ahead and freeze them once cooked.

makes:
10 croquettes

150g cold mashed potato (cooked without salt in the water)
2 spring onions, sliced
25g Parmesan cheese, grated
40g butternut squash, peeled and grated
20g red pepper, finely diced
1 tomato, deseeded and cut into 1cm dice
25g tinned sweetcorn, chopped roughly
1 x 160g tin tuna in sunflower oil, drained
1 egg, beaten
1 tbsp chopped fresh basil
50g panko breadcrumbs
2 tbsp sunflower oil

1. Place the potato, spring onions, Parmesan, squash, red pepper, tomato, sweetcorn, tuna, egg, basil and half of the breadcrumbs into a bowl. Mix well and shape into ten croquettes.

2. Roll the croquettes in the remaining breadcrumbs.

3. Heat the oil in a large non-stick frying pan. Fry the croquettes for 5–8 minutes until golden and heated through.

nutritional benefits
- *Nutritionally complete*
- *Provides vitamin A, vitamin E, vitamin C, iron (combination increases the absorption of iron), iodine and zinc*
- *Source of prebiotics*

198

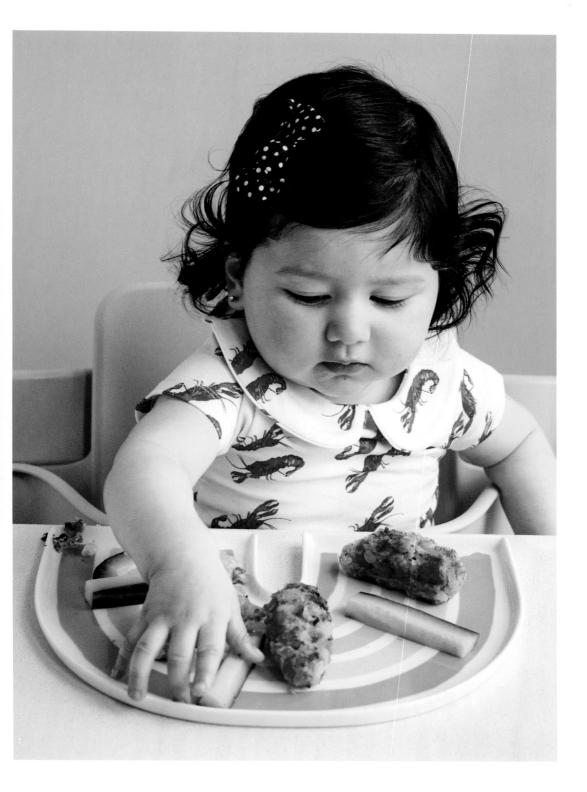

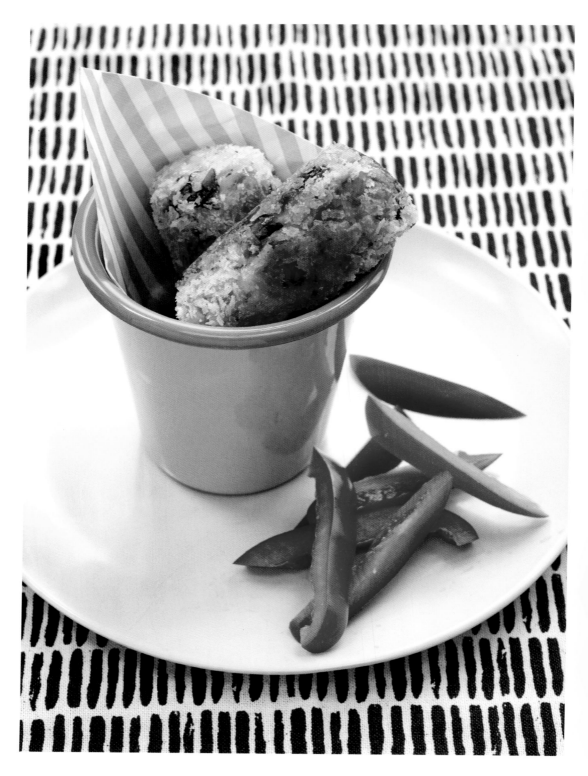

curried fish fingers

These are not your ordinary fish fingers! Cod is coated in a mild curry paste and mango chutney and finished with my special topping. Serve up and win over even the fussiest of eaters! You can also allow to cool and freeze once cooked.

makes:
15 fish fingers

1 tbsp mild curry korma paste
1 tsp mango chutney
2 tbsp plain flour
300g cod loin fillet, all bones removed and sliced into 6cm fingers

50g Rice Krispies
25g Parmesan cheese, finely grated
olive oil, for drizzling

1. Preheat the oven to 220°C (fan 200°C/gas mark 7). Line a baking tray with baking parchment.

2. Mix the curry paste and mango chutney together in a bowl. Place the flour in a separate bowl. Coat the cod fingers in the flour, then dip into the curry and mango mixture.

3. Put the Rice Krispies into a medium bowl and crush with a rolling pin to make fine crumbs. Add the Parmesan cheese and stir to combine.

4. Add the cod to the bowl and coat in the crumbs. Place the fingers on the lined tray and drizzle with olive oil.

5. Bake for 15–18 minutes, until lightly golden and the cod is cooked through.

nutritional benefits
- *Good source of protein*
- *Provides iron, zinc and iodine*

cod cubes with fruity curry sauce

Kids love flavour, fact! And this fruity fish curry will not disappoint. With just the right amount of mild spice and natural sweetness, it's the perfect balance of flavour. Once cooked, you can also allow the cod cubes to cool and freeze them for another day.

makes:
25 cubes

FOR THE SAUCE
1 tsp sunflower oil
1 onion, chopped
50g butternut squash, peeled and grated
¼ eating apple, peeled and grated
1 clove garlic, crushed
½ tsp mild korma curry powder
150ml homemade vegetable stock (see page 105), very low-salt vegetable stock or water
1 tsp mango chutney

FOR THE COD
60g panko breadcrumbs
¼ tsp curry powder
4 tbsp plain flour
1 egg
300g cod loin, all bones removed and cut into 1.5cm
sunflower oil, for drizzling

1. Preheat the oven to 220°C (fan 200°C/gas mark 7). Line a baking tray with baking parchment.

2. To make the curry sauce, heat the oil in a pan. Add the onion, squash and apple and fry for 2–3 minutes.

3. Add the garlic and curry powder and fry for 10 seconds. Add the stock and mango chutney. Cover and simmer for 10 minutes, then blend until smooth.

4. Mix the panko breadcrumbs and curry powder together in a bowl. Place the flour and egg into separate bowls. Beat the egg. Coat the cod cubes in flour. Dip the cubes into the egg, then into the crumb mixture. Shake the bowl to coat the cubes.

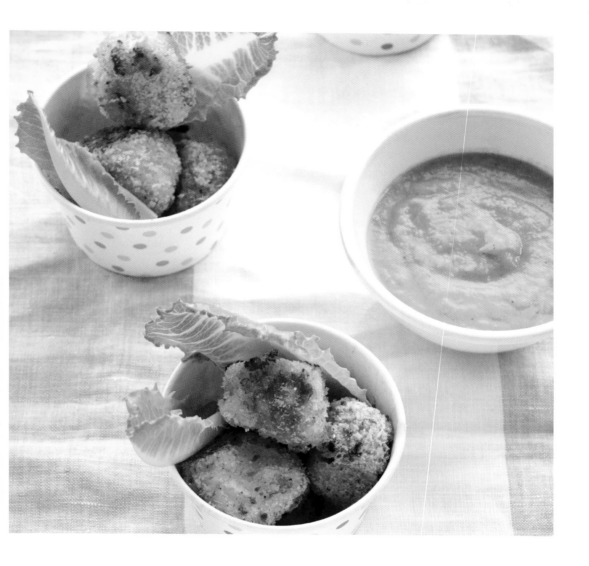

5. Place the coated cubes on a lined or non-stick baking tray and drizzle with oil. Bake for 8–10 minutes, turning over halfway through the cooking time. Serve with the curry sauce.

nutritional benefits

- *Good source of protein*
- *Provides vitamin A, vitamin C, iron (combination increases the absorption of iron), iodine and zinc*
- *Source of prebiotics*

salmon & pea fritters

Fritters are great for kids as you pack them with goodness. These little powerhouses are packed with protein, three different veggies, and provide a good source of omega 3s, vitamin A, vitamin C, calcium, iodine, iron and zinc. Everyone will love tucking into these at the dinner table.

makes:
12 fritters

50g frozen peas
200g boneless salmon fillet
2 eggs
50g butternut squash, peeled and grated

75g courgette, grated
30g plain flour
15g Parmesan cheese, grated (*optional*)
sunflower oil, for frying

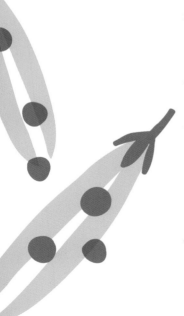

1. Cook the peas in boiling water for 4 minutes, drain and refresh until cold water.

2. Bring a small pan of water up to the boil, Add the salmon fillet, turn down the heat and simmer for 12 minutes until the salmon is cooked. Drain and leave to cool before flaking.

3. Beat the eggs in a bowl. Add the remaining ingredients and stir well.

4. Heat a little oil in a large non-stick frying pan. Add heaped tablespoons of mixture to the pan and fry for 3 minutes on each side, until golden and cooked through. (You may need to cook these in batches.)

nutritional benefits
- *Great source of protein*
- *Provides omega 3s, vitamin A, vitamin C, iron (combination increases the absorption of iron), calcium, iodine and zinc*

haddock, potato & sweetcorn chowder

This simple chowder is a great way to introduce your baby to fish. A cross between a lovely thick and creamy soup and a stew, this hearty recipe makes for the perfect one-pot pleaser for the whole family. Bread at the ready for dipping!

makes:
6 portions

a knob of unsalted butter
1 leek, sliced
1 carrot, peeled and cut into 1cm dice
130g potatoes, peeled and cut into 1cm dice
15g plain flour

200ml very low-salt fish stock
250ml milk
175g haddock or cod fillet, all bones removed and cut into 1.5cm dice
40g tinned sweetcorn
bread, to serve (*optional*)

1. Melt the butter in a pan. Add the leek and carrot and fry for a few minutes. Add the potatoes and flour and fry for 30 seconds. Gradually stir in the fish stock. Bring to the boil, cover and simmer for 8–10 minutes, stirring occasionally.

2. When the potato is nearly soft, add the milk and bring to the boil. Add the haddock and sweetcorn and simmer for 4–5 minutes. Serve with bread, if liked.

nutritional benefits
- *Nutritionally complete*
- *Provides vitamin A, B vitamins, calcium, iodine, iron and zinc*
- *Source of prebiotics*

tuna pasta bake

Who doesn't love a tuna pasta bake? Tinned tuna is a store cupboard essential which packs in protein. And this recipe is also made up of prebiotic foods which will help to stimulate growth of that good bacteria in your baby's gut.

makes:
6 portions

125g macaroni
2 tsp olive oil
75g onions, chopped
50g carrots, peeled and grated
1 clove garlic, crushed
400g tin chopped tomatoes
2 tsp tomato purée

1 tbsp chopped fresh basil or
  1 tsp dried basil
1 tbsp cream cheese
50g tinned sweetcorn
50g peas
100g tinned tuna
60g Cheddar cheese, grated

1. Preheat the oven to 220°C (fan 200°C/gas mark 7).

2. Cook the macaroni according to the packet instructions. Drain.

3. Heat the oil in a pan. Add the onions and carrots and fry for 5 minutes. Add the garlic and cook for 30 seconds.

4. Add the tomatoes and tomato purée and simmer for 20 minutes. Stir in the basil and cream cheese. Blend until smooth.

5. Add the pasta, sweetcorn, peas and tuna and mix well, to combine. Spoon into 6 ramekins and sprinkle with cheese. Bake for 15–20 minutes.

nutritional benefits
- *Nutritionally complete*
- *Provides vitamin A, vitamin C, iron (combination increases the absorption of iron), calcium, magnesium, iodine and zinc*
- *Source of prebiotics*

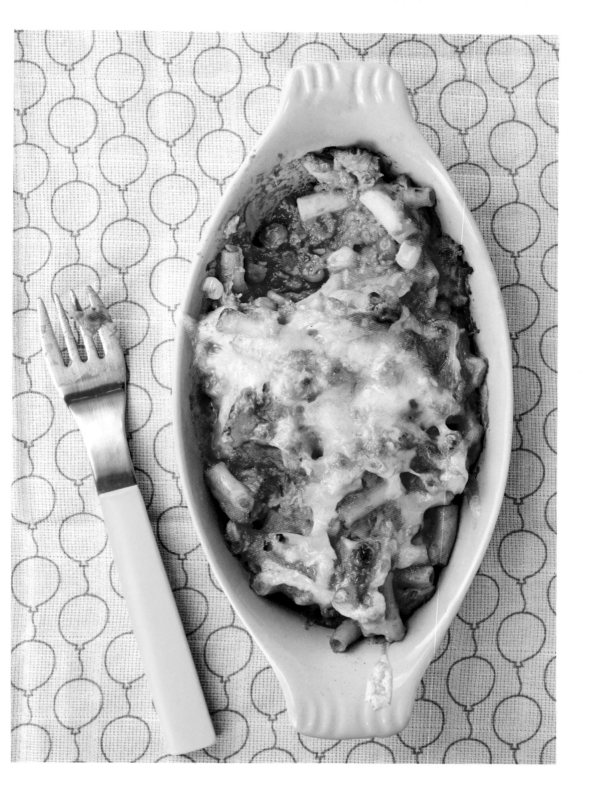

salmon with pasta shells

We know that salmon is full of essential goodness and pairing it with something little ones love, such as pasta, is a great way to ensure it ends up in their tummies rather than on the floor! Baking the salmon in a foil parcel makes it soft and the butternut squash adds a natural sweetness.

makes:
5 portions

100g salmon fillet, skinned and all bones removed
a knob of unsalted butter
50g mini pasta shells
85g butternut squash, peeled and diced into tiny pieces
60g small broccoli florets
2 tomatoes, deseeded, skinned and chopped
20g Parmesan cheese, grated

1. Preheat the oven to 180°C (fan 160°C/gas mark 4). Place the salmon on a piece of foil, top with half the butter, and fold over the edges to seal. Place on a baking tray.

2. Bake for 12 minutes until cooked. Flake the fish and leave to cool. Cook the pasta according to the packet instructions. Drain.

3. Place the squash in the lower level of a multi layered steamer, place the broccoli in the top level of the steamer and steam the vegetables for 7 minutes until tender.

4. Melt the remaining butter in a pan, add the tomatoes and cook for a few seconds, then add the salmon and juices, vegetables and cheese and mix well.

nutritional benefits
- *Nutritionally complete*
- *Provides omega 3s, vitamin A, vitamin C, iron (combination increases the absorption of iron), calcium, iodine and zinc*
- *Source of prebiotics*

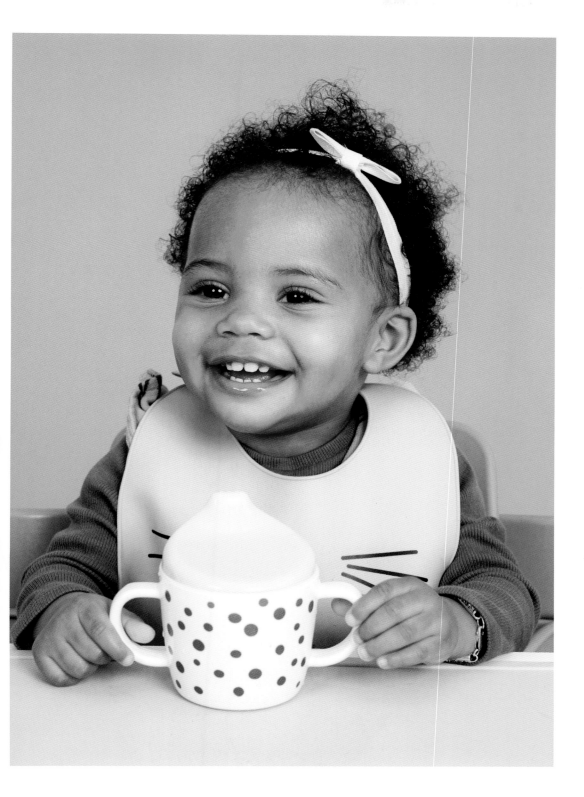

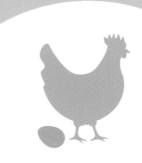

9–12 months
poultry

turkey burgers

My nutritious turkey burgers make for a great finger food for babies. Serve in soft buns and some roasted sweet potato wedges and you have a feast for the whole family. These are also ideal for batch freezing.

makes:
15 mini burgers

350g minced turkey thigh
½ eating apple, peeled and grated
1 small carrot, peeled and grated
¼ red pepper, finely chopped

1 tbsp chopped fresh sage
30g Cheddar cheese, grated
45g panko breadcrumbs
oil, for frying

1. Place all the ingredients into a food processor. Whiz until finely chopped. Shape into fifteen mini burgers.

2. Heat a little sunflower oil in a large non-stick frying pan. Fry the burgers for 2–3 minutes on each side, until golden and cooked through. (You may need to cook in batches.)

nutritional benefits
- *Good source of protein*
- *Provides vitamin C, selenium, iron and zinc*

roast chicken

My whole family love this roast chicken recipe, and it's simple to prepare. Pop everything onto two baking trays and then cook in the oven for 25–30 minutes. Either cut up the roasted chicken and vegetables into manageable slices for your baby or blend to a purée (see page 214).

If you have any leftovers try my tortilla chicken cups (see page 215), curried chicken & veggie croquettes (see page 217), or gnocchi with chicken, tomato & basil (see page 218).

roast chicken with sweet potato, thyme & peppers

makes:
4 adult portions
plus baby

1 x 1.5kg chicken, jointed
1 clove garlic, crushed
1 tbsp chopped fresh thyme, chopped
3 tbsp olive oil

3 sweet potatoes, peeled and cut into 1.5cm cubes
2 banana shallots, sliced
1 red pepper, cut into 1.5cm pieces

1. Preheat the oven to 220°C (fan 200°C/gas mark 7).

2. Put the chicken breasts, thighs and drumsticks into a bowl. Add the garlic, thyme and 1 tablespoon of the oil. Toss to coat.

3. Divide the sweet potato, shallots and peppers between two baking trays. Drizzle with the remaining 2 tablespoons oil.

CONTINUED OVERLEAF

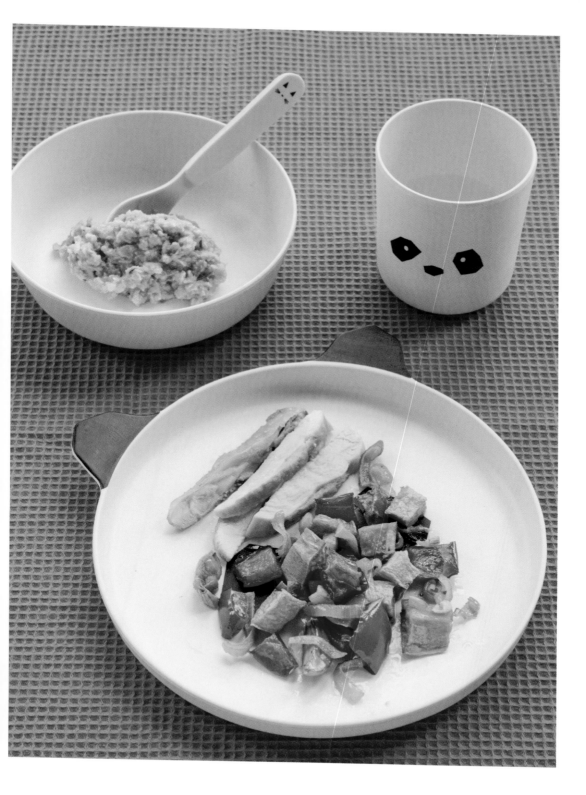

4. Put the chicken breasts and drumsticks on top of the vegetables on one tray. Put the chicken thighs on top of the vegetables on the other baking tray.

5. Roast the chicken and vegetables for 25–30 minutes or until the chicken is cooked and golden and the juices run clear and the vegetables are brown and soft.

6. Serve the chicken with the roasted vegetables, chopping up a small portion of everything for your baby.

MAKE WITH YOUR LEFTOVERS There is no reason your baby can't enjoy the same meal as a purée. This recipe shows you how to adapt the adult recipe easily and quickly so she can join you at mealtimes.

roast chicken dinner purée

makes:
2–3 baby portions

meat from 1 roasted chicken thigh
100g mixed roasted vegetables

1. Put the chicken and vegetables into a food processor and whiz until smooth.

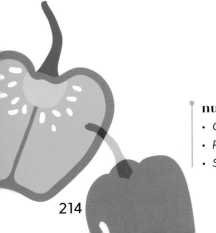

nutritional benefits

- *Good source of protein*
- *Provides vitamin A, selenium, iron and zinc*
- *Source of prebiotics*

MAKE WITH YOUR LEFTOVERS

Tortilla wraps are a quick, easy and lighter alternative to pastry and make the perfect 'cups' for delicious fillings. I've used chicken, cherry tomatoes, sweetcorn and cheese here but feel free to tweak the fillings depending on what you have to hand.

tortilla chicken cups

makes:
6 cups

You will also need:
6-hole muffin tin

sunflower oil, for brushing
6 mini tortilla wraps
25g unsalted butter
25g plain flour
250ml milk
75g tinned sweetcorn

125g cooked chicken, cut into 1cm dice
25g Parmesan cheese, grated
4 cherry tomatoes, quartered
2 tbsp chopped fresh basil
25g Cheddar cheese, grated

1. Preheat the oven to 180°C (fan 160°C/gas mark 4). Brush the hollows of the muffin tin with oil. Trim the tortilla wraps to 14 cm diameter. Line the muffin tin with the wraps, pushing them into the holes. These will form the shells for the chicken filling.

2. Melt the butter in a pan. Add the flour. Whisk for 30 seconds. Whisk in the milk. Bring up to the boil, whisking until thickened. Remove from the heat.

3. Stir in the sweetcorn, chicken, Parmesan, tomatoes and basil.

4. Spoon the mixture into the cups and sprinkle with grated Cheddar. Bake for 18–20 minutes until golden.

nutritional benefits
- *Nutritionally complete*
- *Provides vitamin C, iron (combination increases the absorption of iron), calcium and zinc*
- *Source of prebiotics*

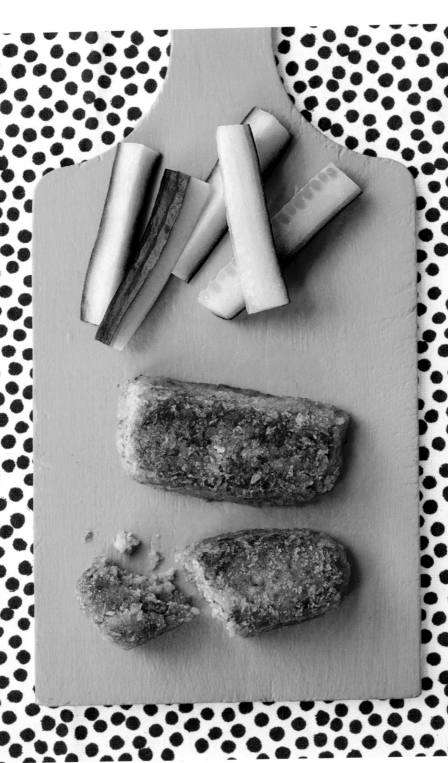

MAKE WITH YOUR LEFTOVERS

Ever wondered what to do with leftover roast chicken? Try these mildly spiced croquettes – crunchy on the outside and succulent on the inside. They are loaded with lots of essential nutrients and are easy to freeze.

curried chicken & veggie croquettes

makes:
8 croquettes

30g small broccoli florets
125g cold mashed potato (cooked without salt in the water)
60g carrot, peeled and grated
4 spring onions, thinly sliced
80g cooked chicken, diced
50g tinned chickpeas

1 tsp curry powder
½ tsp mango chutney
20g Parmesan cheese, grated
1 egg
30g panko breadcrumbs
sunflower oil, for frying

1. Steam the broccoli for 3 minutes. Refresh under cold water, then roughly chop.

2. Place the broccoli, potato, carrot, onions, chicken, chickpeas, curry powder, mango chutney and cheese together in a food processor. Whiz until finely chopped. Shape into eight croquettes.

3. Place the egg in a bowl and beat. Place the breadcrumbs in a separate bowl. Dip each croquette in the beaten egg and then roll in the panko breadcrumbs. Chill in the fridge for 30 minutes.

4. Heat the oil in a large non-stick frying pan. Fry the croquettes, for 8 minutes, turning occasionally, until golden brown and crisp.

nutritional benefits
- *Nutritionally complete*
- *Provides vitamin A, vitamin C, iron (combination increases the absorption of iron) and zinc*
- *Source of prebiotics*

MAKE WITH YOUR LEFTOVERS

Gnocchi is a great alternative to pasta, and this recipe provides a concentrated source of energy that will help to fuel growth in your baby's first year. The cheese and cream also provide all-important calcium to their diet which is essential for strong bones.

gnocchi with chicken, tomato & basil

makes:
5 portions

250g fresh gnocchi
1 tbsp olive oil
1 shallot, diced
1 small clove garlic, crushed
3 tbsp double cream

220g cherry tomatoes, halved
120g cooked chicken, diced
25g Parmesan cheese, grated
a squeeze of lemon juice
1 heaped tbsp chopped fresh basil

1. Cook the gnocchi according to the packet instructions. Drain, reserving 3 tablespoons of the cooking water.

2. Heat the oil in a frying pan or pan. Add the shallot and sauté for 5 minutes.

3. Add the garlic and sauté for 30 seconds. Add the cream and the reserved gnocchi cooking water and bring up to the boil.

4. Add the tomatoes and chicken and cook over a low heat for 2 minutes, then remove from the heat and stir in the Parmesan, lemon and basil. Stir through the gnocchi and serve.

nutritional benefits
- *Nutritionally complete*
- *Provides vitamin C, iron (combination increases the absorption of iron) and zinc*
- *Source of prebiotics*

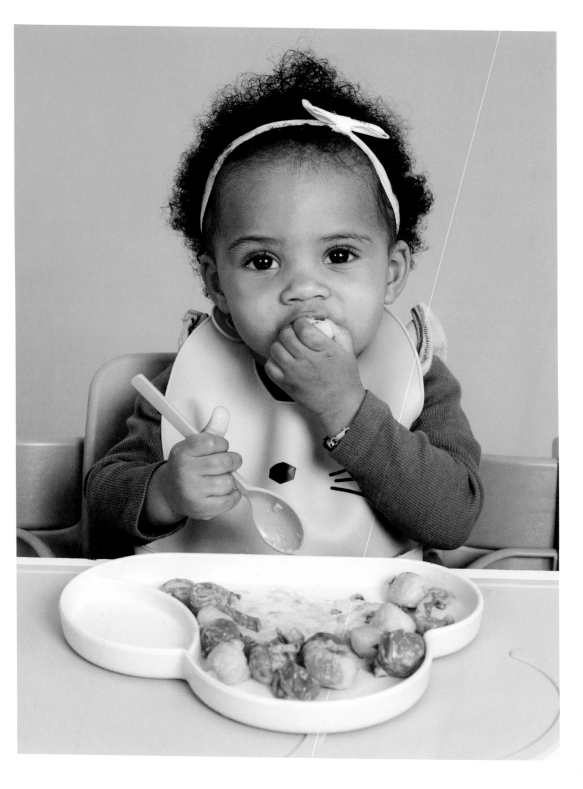

herby chicken goujons with tomato & basil sauce

This is my healthy, tasty take on shop-bought chicken nuggets. Flavoured with herbs and a little Parmesan, my goujons are a fantastic source of protein for your growing baby.

You'll only need to serve half the quantity of tomato sauce with the goujons. Use the remaining sauce in other recipes such as tuna pasta bake (see page 206) or any of my meatball recipes. Alternatively freeze it so you have a ready-to-go sauce for those busy days when you need dinner in a flash.

makes:
10 goujons

FOR THE SAUCE
1 tbsp olive oil
2 onions, chopped
1 carrot, peeled and grated
1 clove garlic, crushed
2 x 400g cans chopped tomatoes
1 tbsp tomato purée
2 tbsp chopped fresh basil

FOR THE GOUJONS
a handful of fresh basil and
    parsley leaves
½ clove garlic, crushed
2 slices of white bread
2 tbsp finely grated Parmesan
    cheese
1 egg
50g plain flour
2 skinless chicken breasts, each
    sliced into 5 strips
sunflower oil, for drizzling

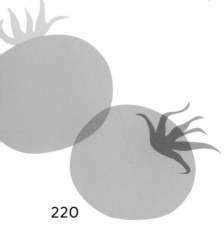

1. To make the tomato sauce, heat the oil in a pan. Add the onions and carrot and fry for 3-4 minutes. Add the garlic and fry for 30 seconds. Mix in the tomatoes and tomato purée. Bring to the boil, cover and simmer for 20 minutes. Stir in the basil, then blend until smooth.

2. Preheat the oven to 230°C (fan 210°C/gas mark 8). Line a baking tray with baking parchment.

3. Put the herbs and garlic into a food processor whiz until chopped, then add the bread and Parmesan. Whiz until finely chopped. Tip onto a plate.

4. Place the egg in a bowl and beat. Place the flour in a separate bowl. Coat the chicken in the flour, then dip into the beaten egg and then into the breadcrumbs. Arrange the goujons on the lined tray. Drizzle with oil.

5. Bake for 12–15 minutes until lightly golden and cooked through. Serve the goujons with half the tomato sauce.

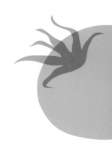

nutritional benefits
- *Good source of protein*
- *Provides vitamin A, vitamin C, iron (combination increases the absorption of iron), selenium and zinc*
- *Source of prebiotics*

turkey, apple & cranberry balls

Christmas or not, your little one will want to devour these bite-sized little gems all year round. You can also freeze them once cooked.

makes:
24 turkey balls

1 small onion, chopped
250g minced turkey thigh
1 eating apple, peeled and diced
25g dried cranberries, chopped
30g panko breadcrumbs
25g Parmesan cheese, grated

1 small egg, beaten
1 tsp chopped fresh thyme
1 tsp dried oregano
2 tbsp plain flour
sunflower oil, for frying

1. Place all the ingredients, except the flour, into a food processor. Whiz together until finely chopped. Shape into 24 meatballs. Place the flour in a bowl. Roll the meatballs in flour, to coat.

2. Heat a little oil in a large non-stick frying pan. Add the meatballs and fry until golden on all sides and cooked through, about 8–10 minutes.

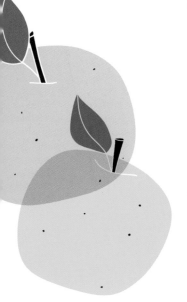

nutritional benefits
- *Good source of protein*
- *Provides vitamin C, iron (combination increases the absorption of iron), calcium and zinc*
- *Source of prebiotics*

cherub's chicken & vegetable curry

There is no reason why little ones can't join in on curry nights too! It's so important to introduce flavours like this to your baby early on.

makes:
6 portions

1 tbsp sunflower oil
200g chicken breast, cut into
  1.5cm dice
1 onion, chopped
2 small carrots, peeled and cut into
  1cm dice
1 clove garlic, crushed
2 tsp korma curry paste

½–1 tsp garam masala
2 tsp tomato purée
1 x 225g tin chopped tomatoes
400ml tin full-fat coconut milk
30g frozen peas
½ tsp mango chutney (*optional*)
rice, to serve (*optional*)

1. Heat the oil in a frying pan. Add the chicken and fry until sealed.

2. Add the onion and carrots and fry for 2 minutes. Add the garlic, curry paste, garam masala, tomato purée and fresh tomatoes. Simmer for 3 minutes.

3. Stir in the coconut milk. Bring to the boil, then reduce the heat and simmer for 10 minutes, until the sauce has thickened slightly.

4. Mix in the peas and mango chutney, if using.

5. Simmer for 4 minutes or until the peas and chicken are cooked through. Serve with rice, if liked.

nutritional benefits
- *Good source of protein*
- *Provides vitamin A, vitamin C, iron (combination increases the absorption of iron) and zinc*
- *Source of prebiotics*

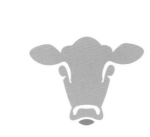

9–12 months
beef

roast beef

Sunday lunch is a big deal, which is why baby should enjoy a piece of the action – after all, it's all about coming together at the dinner table. My delicious beef paired with roast white and sweet potatoes and veggies is a well-balanced meal for your youngest family member. You can make the beef croquettes and mini yorkshires with roast beef with the leftovers.

makes:
6 adult portions
plus baby

1.8kg trimmed beef topside
5 tbsp olive oil
2 tbsp chopped fresh sage
2 tbsp chopped fresh thyme
1 bulb garlic, halved
salt and pepper
800g white potatoes, peeled and
   cut into chunks
600g sweet potatoes, peeled and
   cut into chunks

steamed peas and carrots, to serve

FOR THE GRAVY
3 tbsp plain flour
2 tsp tomato purée
150ml red wine (optional, if not
   using increase stock to 600ml)
450ml very low-salt beef stock (or
   600ml, see above)

1. Preheat the oven to 230°C (fan 210°C/gas mark 8).

2. Rub the beef with 1 tablespoon of the oil, the sage and half the thyme and place in a roasting tin with the halved garlic bulb. Season the beef, then roast for 10 minutes. Reduce the oven temperature to 220°C (fan 200°C/gas mark 7) and roast for 50–60 minutes. Cover with tin foil and set aside to rest.

3. While the beef is resting, divide the remaining oil between two baking trays and place in the oven to heat.

4. Bring a pan of water to the boil, add the white and sweet potato and parboil for 5 minutes. Drain, then add the potatoes to the two baking trays and roast for 30–35 minutes, turning halfway through, until crisp and brown. Scatter the remaining thyme on top.

CONTINUED OVERLEAF

5. Remove the beef from the roasting tin and set aside on a warmed plate. Cover with foil. Stir the flour into the leftover cooking juices in the tin, and whisk until smooth.

6. Place the roasting tin on the hob. Add the tomato purée, wine (if using) and stock, whisk and bring to the boil. Serve the gravy with the beef and plate up with the veg, chopping up a small portion of everything for your baby.

MAKE WITH YOUR LEFTOVERS

There's nothing more satisfying than transforming leftovers into a dish equally as delicious as the main event. Using leftover roast beef and potatoes, my beef croquettes contain all the same goodness as your roast dinner but in finger food form. You can also freeze them once cooked.

roast beef croquettes

makes:
8 croquettes

175g cold mashed potato (cooked without salt in the water)
3 spring onions, finely chopped
50g cooked beef, diced
1 small carrot, peeled and grated

20g Parmesan cheese, grated
2 tbsp mayonnaise
4 tbsp plain flour
sunflower oil, for frying

1. Mix all of the ingredients, except the flour, together in a bowl. Shape the mixture into 8 sausage shapes. Place the flour in a bowl. Roll the croquettes in the flour, to coat.

2. Heat a little oil in a large non-stick frying pan. Fry the sausages for 3–4 minutes on each side until golden and cooked through.

nutritional benefits
- *Nutritionally complete*
- *Provides vitamin A, vitamin C, iron (combination increases the absorption of iron) and zinc*
- *Source of prebiotics*

Another of my beef leftover favourites! My mini Yorkshire puddings are just like a roast dinner canapé and intriguing for little hands. You'll have some batter left over which you can make into more Yorkshire puddings or pancakes (both freeze well).

mini yorkshire puddings with roast beef

makes:
24 puddings

. . . .

You will also need:
24-hole mini
muffin tin

50g plain flour
1 large egg
100ml milk

sunflower oil, for oiling
2 tbsp shop-bought mayonnaise
100g cooked roast beef, sliced

1. Preheat the oven to 230°C (fan 210°C/gas mark 8).

2. To make the batter, place the flour, eggs, and milk into a bowl. Whisk until smooth. Pour the batter into a clean empty squeezy bottle (an empty ketchup bottle works well).

3. Pour a little oil into the muffin holes in the tin. Place in the oven for 5 minutes to heat.

4. Squeeze a little batter into each muffin hole, about one quarter of the way up the sides of each one. Cook for 10–12 minutes, until well risen, golden and crisp. Remove the puddings from the tin and leave to cool a little on a wire rack.

5. Spoon a little mayonnaise into the base of each pudding. Slice the beef and arrange inside the puddings.

nutritional benefits

- *Good source of protein*
- *Provides vitamin D, calcium, iron and zinc*
- *Source of prebiotics*

mini cottage pies

At this stage your baby will be able to eat lots of what your family is having (just without any added salt). Serve up their own individual portions and let them join in at mealtimes.

makes:
2 pies

....

You will also need
2 x 150ml ramekins
(*or 3 smaller ramekins if you prefer*)

1 tbsp olive oil
1 onion, chopped
1 small carrot, peeled and cut into 1cm dice
¼ red pepper, cut into 1cm dice
8 button mushrooms, cut into 1cm dice
250g minced beef
1 tbsp tomato purée

1 tbsp plain flour
250ml very low-salt beef stock
2 dried bay leaves
1 tsp chopped fresh thyme
300g potatoes, peeled and chopped into 2cm pieces
a knob of unsalted butter
1–2 tbsp milk

1. Preheat the oven to 200°C (fan 180°C/gas mark 6).

2. Heat the oil in a pan. Add the onion, carrot, pepper and mushrooms and fry for 3–4 minutes.

3. Add the mince and brown. Stir in the tomato purée and flour, then blend in the stock and add the bay leaves and thyme. Cover and simmer for 30 minutes over a low heat. Spoon into two ramekins, discarding the bay leaves.

4. For the mash, bring a pan of water to the boil, add the potatoes and boil for 15 minutes or until tender. Drain, mash and mix with the butter and milk. Divide the mash between the ramekins, spreading it out to cover the filling. Bake the pies for 15 minutes.

nutritional benefits

- *Nutritionally complete*
- *Provides vitamin A, calcium, zinc and iron*
- *Source of prebiotics*

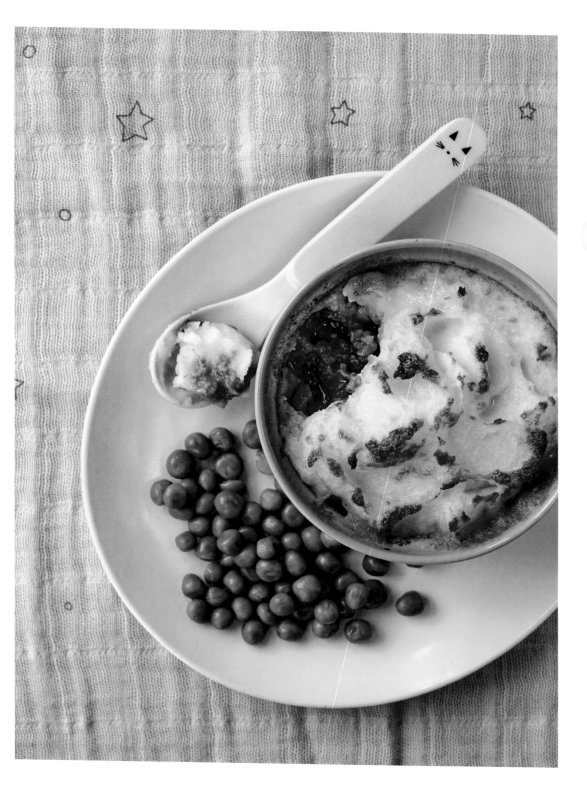

2-IN-1 RECIPE

Whizzing beef in a blender helps babies to tackle its texture. It is so easy to adapt this recipe to make meatballs. Serve them with a tomato sauce to make a complete meal for the whole family.

THE PURÉE

butternut squash, red onion & pepper purée

makes:
4 portions

250g butternut squash, peeled and cut into 1.5cm dice
1 red onion, sliced
1 small red pepper, cut into 1.5cm dice
2 tbsp sunflower oil
250g lean minced beef
2 tsp chopped fresh thyme

1. Preheat the oven to 220°C (fan 200°C/gas mark 7).

2. Put the squash, onion and pepper onto a baking tray. Toss in the oil, to coat, and roast for 25 minutes. Transfer to a bowl.

3. Heat a frying pan over a high heat. Add the beef and brown it.

4. Add the beef to the bowl with the vegetables. Blend with an electric stick blender, gradually adding up to 200ml boiling water, to the desired consistency. Stir in the thyme.

FINGER FOOD

butternut squash, red onion & pepper mini meatballs

makes:
25 balls

Same ingredients as listed left with the addition of:
extra oil, for frying
30g panko breadcrumbs

1. Bake the vegetables as described in step 1 of the purée, left. Leave to cool, then add to the food processer with the thyme, breadcrumbs and beef and whiz until finely chopped. Shape into twenty-five balls.

2. Heat a little oil in a large non-stick frying pan. Add the balls and fry over a medium heat for 10 minutes, until cooked through and browned. You can also allow to cool and freeze for another day.

nutritional benefits of both
- *Good source of protein*
- *Provides zinc, vitamin A, vitamin C, iron (combination increases absorption of iron)*
- *Source of prebiotics*

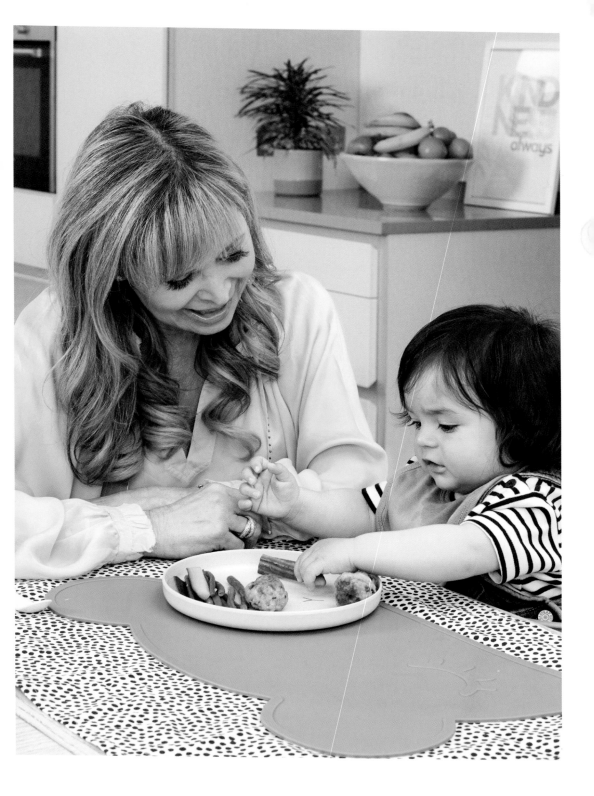

bolognese pasta bake

Waste not, want not! Use any leftover mini cottage pie meat mixture to cook up this baby favourite.

makes:
2 portions

75g mini pasta shells
40g frozen peas
½ quantity of mini cottage pie meat mixture (see page 228)

25g mature Cheddar cheese, grated

1. Preheat the grill to high.

2. Cook the pasta according to the packet instructions, adding the peas 3 minutes before the end of the cooking time. Drain. Meanwhile, heat the meat mixture in a small saucepan over a medium heat until hot.

3. Mix the warmed mini cottage pie mixture into the pasta. Stir in half the cheese.

4. Spoon the pasta and meat into two ramekins and sprinkle with the remaining cheese. Place under a hot grill for 5 minutes.

nutritional benefits
- *Nutritionally complete*
- *Provides vitamin A, vitamin C, iron (combination increases the absorption of iron), calcium and zinc*

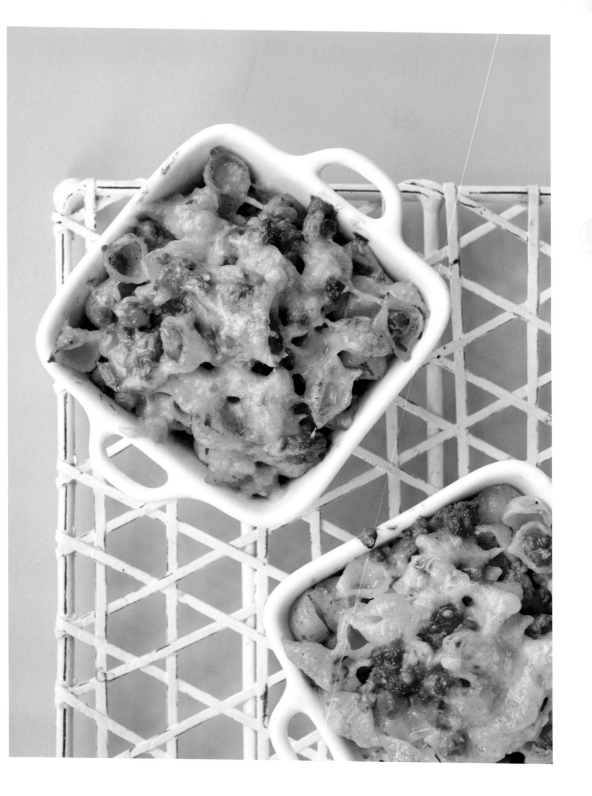

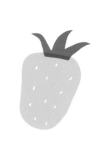

9–12 months
snacks

chicken, cucumber & cheese straws

Weaning is a sensory experience and so if you can, try to make their food not only taste good but look good too. Something as simple as threading colourful food onto a straw will keep little hands and mouths busy!

makes:
3 straws

. . . .

You will also need
metal skewer
3 paper straws

1 large slice of Edam cheese
1 slice of ciabatta bread
½ cooked chicken breast

¼ cucumber
3 cherry tomatoes, halved

1. Slice the cheese into six strips. Cut the bread into six cubes. Slice the chicken into five bite-sized pieces and peel the cucumber into six ribbons, using a vegetable peeler. Halve the tomatoes.

2. Thread a cube of bread, then a piece of cheese, then cucumber, chicken and half a cherry tomato onto a skewer to make holes. Transfer to a paper straw and repeat.

nutritional benefits
- *Nutritionally complete*
- *Provides vitamin C, , iron (combination increases the absorption of iron) calcium, iodine and zinc*

yoghurt-based pizza margherita

A fast-food favourite but not as you know it! I recently discovered that just two ingredients – Greek yoghurt and self-raising flour – make the perfect pizza base. Combine this with my special homemade tomato sauce, and you have the perfect snack – or you can also serve the whole pizza as a meal. Bellissimo!

makes:
4 small pizzas

150g self-raising flour plus extra for dusting
125g Greek yoghurt
100g passata
1 tsp sundried tomato purée
2 tbsp chopped fresh basil

8 cherry tomatoes, sliced
75g mature Cheddar cheese, grated
75g mozzarella cheese, diced
1 tsp chopped fresh thyme

1. Preheat the oven to 220°C (fan 200°C/gas mark 7). Line two baking trays with baking parchment.

2. Place the flour and yoghurt into a bowl. Mix well and stir into a dough. Knead on a floured work surface until smooth. Divide the dough into four equal pieces on a floured surface. Roll it out to make four 12cm bases. Place on the baking trays.

3. Mix the passata, sundried tomato purée and basil together in a bowl. Spoon on top of the bases and spread out. Top with the sliced tomatoes, cheeses and thyme.

4. Bake for 15 minutes until golden on top and underneath. Cut into quarters and serve a slice as a snack. Allow the other slices to cool and freeze in a plastic box separated by greaseproof paper.

nutritional benefits
- *Nutritionally complete*
- *Provides vitamin C, iron (combination increases the absorption of iron) and calcium*
- *Source of prebiotics*

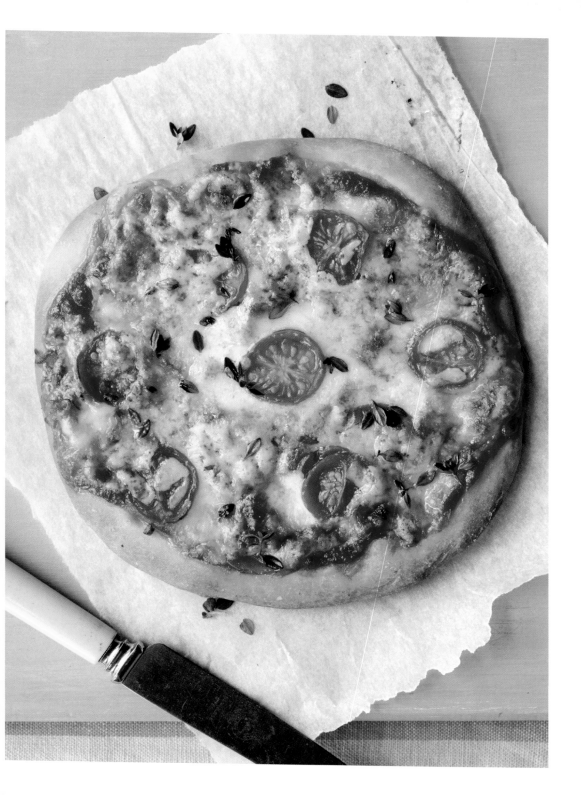

pitta & veggie platter with guacamole dip

This nutritious platter will allow little ones to dunk and dip with glee.

makes:
6 child portions

3 pitta breads, halved through the middle
2 tbsp fresh pesto
2 tbsp grated Parmesan cheese
1 carrot, peeled and sliced into batons
1 red pepper, deseeded and sliced into strips
1 cucumber, sliced into strips

FOR THE DIP
1 avocado, halved, pitted, peeled and sliced
3 cherry tomatoes, halved
juice of ¼ lemon
¼ clove garlic, crushed
2 tbsp Greek yoghurt

1. Brush the pitta bread with pesto and sprinkle with the Parmesan cheese. Place on a baking tray. Grill for 5–7 minutes until golden and crisp. Leave to cool, then slice into strips horizontally.

2. Place all the dip ingredients in a food processor. Whiz until smooth. Serve it with the vegetable sticks and pitta strips.

nutritional benefits
• *Provides vitamin C*

soured cream & herb dip

This dip is a good source of protein, vitamin A and calcium and is delicious served on toast, pitta, or oat cakes with a selection of vegetable sticks.

makes:
6 portions

150g soured cream
50g Greek yoghurt
180g cream cheese
2 tbsp grated Parmesan cheese
½ clove garlic, crushed
2 spring onions, chopped
6 fresh basil leaves, chopped
2 tsp chopped fresh chives
toast, pitta or oat cakes and vegetable sticks,
  to serve

1. Place the sour cream, yoghurt, cream cheese, Parmesan cheese, garlic and spring onions into a food processor. Whiz until smooth.

2. Add the basil and chives and pulse until chopped. Serve with toast, pitta or oat cakes and vegetable sticks.

nutritional benefits
• *Good source of protein*
• *Provides vitamin A, calcium and iodine*
• *Source of prebiotics*

broccoli & cheese muffins

Superfood muffins you say? If you're looking for new ways to 'super-fy' your baby's snacks then look no further than my broccoli muffins – they're packed with vitamins A, C and D. You can also freeze these when cooked.

makes:
12 muffins

. . . .

You will also need
12-hole silicone
muffin tray

75g broccoli florets
225g self-raising flour
1 tsp baking powder
1 tbsp chopped fresh chives
50g Cheddar cheese, grated

40g Parmesan cheese, grated
4 cherry tomatoes, quartered
2 eggs
200ml buttermilk
75ml sunflower oil

1. Preheat the oven to 180°C (fan 160°C/gas mark 4).

2. Steam the broccoli for 4 minutes. Chop or mash and leave to cool.

3. Mix the flour, baking powder, chives and cheeses together in a large bowl.

4. Mix the eggs, buttermilk and oil together. Add the wet ingredients to the dry. Mix together and fold in the broccoli and tomatoes.

5. Spoon the mixture into the muffin tray moulds. Place the tray on a baking tray. Bake for 25–30 minutes, until well risen and lightly golden. Allow to cool for 5 minutes before turning out and cooling on a wire rack. They keep in a plastic container in the fridge for up to 3 days.

nutritional benefits
· *Provides vitamin A, vitamin C, vitamin D, calcium and iodine*
· *Source of prebiotics*

banana & peanut butter sushi

Sushi for babies? Sure! This recipe makes for a fantastic snack for fussy eaters!

makes:
12 sushi pieces

2 mini tortilla wraps

2 tbsp smooth peanut butter

2 tsp chia seeds

2 bananas

1. Put the wraps onto a board. Spread with peanut butter. Sprinkle over the chia seeds. Trim the bananas to fit the wraps and then peel.

2. Place a banana on one side of each wrap and roll up. Slice each wrap into six.

nutritional benefits
- *Nutritionally complete*
- *Provides vitamin C and iron (combination increases the absorption of iron)*
- *Source of prebiotics*

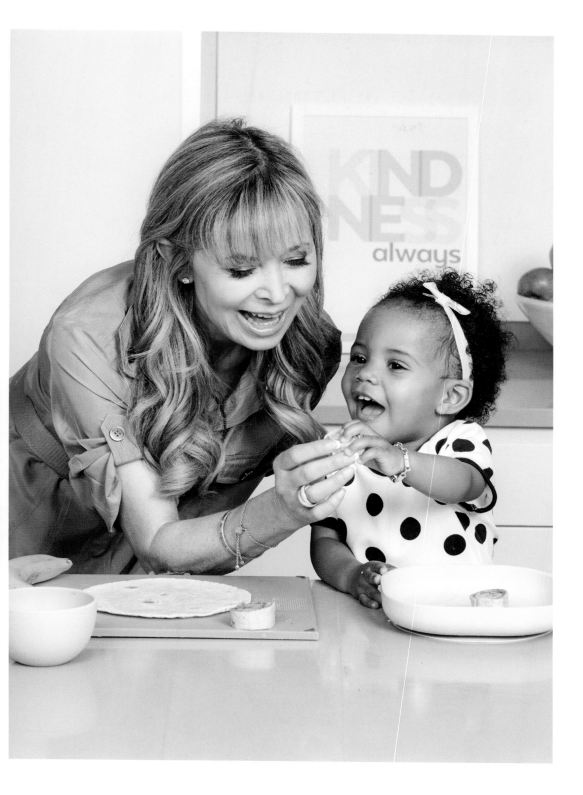

oat, apple & banana bites

These soft baked mini fruity bites are perfect for self-feeding and make a great snack or breakfast.

makes:
18 bites

200g overripe bananas, mashed
1 egg, beaten
120g porridge oats
1 tbsp chia seeds

a pinch of mixed spice
50g dried apple, finely diced
20g sultanas

1. Preheat the oven to 200°C (fan 180°C/gas mark 6). Line a baking tray with baking parchment.

2. Mix the banana and egg together in a bowl. Add the remaining ingredients and beat together.

3. Roll the mixture into eighteen balls and place on the lined tray. Press down slightly. Bake for 10 minutes. You can store these in a tin for up to 3 days.

nutritional benefits

- *Nutritionally complete*
- *Provides vitamin A and vitamin C*
- *Source of prebiotics*

energy balls with peanut butter

Research suggests that babies are less likely to develop allergies if they are introduced to certain foods early on – peanuts and tree nuts being top of the list. The peanut butter and grounded pecans pack a protein punch here, and the oats will give your baby slow release energy. The perfect way to fuel play.

makes:
15–20 balls

150g dates
2 tbsp smooth peanut butter
75g porridge oats
20g Rice Krispies
25g pecan nuts
25g desiccated coconut

1 tbsp chia seeds
10g pumpkin seeds
2 tbsp sunflower oil
a pinch of mixed spice

1. Put the dates and 75ml water into a pan. Cover and bring to the boil. Leave to stand for 5 minutes. Tip the dates and cooking liquid into a food processor and blend until smooth.

2. Chop the pecans in a food processor, add the oats, Rice Krispies, desiccated coconut and chia seeds and pulse for a few seconds. Add the peanut butter, sunflower oil, mixed spice and date purée and whiz the mixture in the food processor until blended.

3. Roll into 15–20 balls and chill in the fridge for at least 1 hour. Keep stored in the fridge.

nutritional benefits
- *Nutritionally complete*
- *Provides vitamin C and iron (combination increases the absorption of iron)*
- *Source of prebiotics*

243

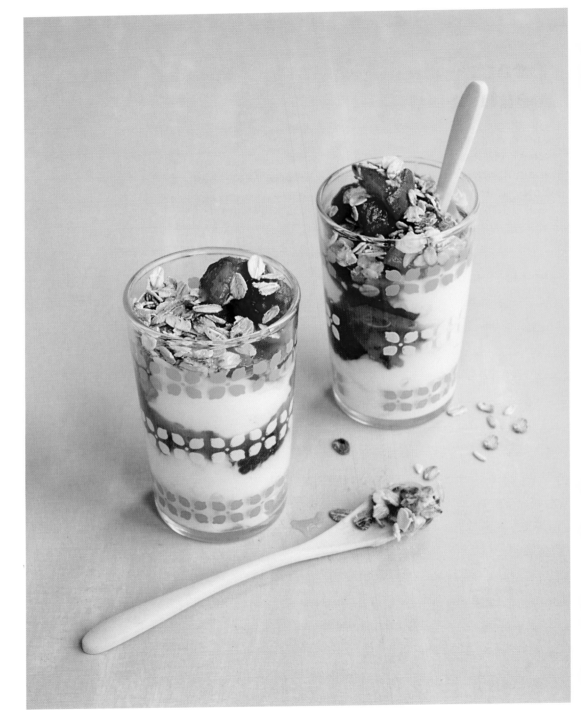

peach & raspberry yoghurt pots

These yummy pots have it all – sweet fruit blended with Greek yoghurt and a sprinkling of oats. It's also high on the nutritious scale too, containing vitamins C and E, calcium and iron. If you're using very ripe peaches, they will only need to be cooked for a couple of minutes.

makes:
2–3 portions

a knob of unsalted butter
2 ripe peaches, diced
1 tsp maple syrup
100g raspberries

4 tbsp porridge oats
200g Greek yoghurt
1 tsp pure vanilla extract
maple syrup, to taste

1. Melt the butter in a pan. Add the peaches and cook gently for 3–5 minutes until just softened. Add the maple syrup. Remove from the heat. Add the raspberries and leave to cool down.

2. Put the oats in a frying pan. Toast over the heat for 2–3 minutes until lightly golden. Leave to cool.

3. Spoon half the yoghurt mixture into two bowls. Spoon half the fruits on top, then the remaining yoghurt and the remaining fruits. Sprinkle with oats and drizzle with maple syrup, to taste.

nutritional benefits
- *Nutritionally complete*
- *Provides vitamin E, vitamin C, iron (combination increases the absorption of iron) and calcium*
- *Source of prebiotics*

apple & blueberry mini muffins

This is a very simple muffin recipe and adding a little mixed spice is a tasty way to introduce your baby to new flavours.

makes:
24 muffins

....

You will also need
24 hole mini muffin tin and paper mini muffin cases

50g unsalted butter, at room temperature
60g caster sugar
60g natural yoghurt
1 tsp pure vanilla extract
110g self-raising flour

1 tsp baking powder
¼ tsp bicarbonate of soda
½ eating apple, peeled and grated
1 tsp mixed spice
100g blueberries

1. Preheat the oven to 180°C (fan 160°C/gas mark 4). Line the tin with the paper cases.

2. Place all the ingredients, except the blueberries, into a bowl. Whisk until smooth, using an electric hand-held whisk. Stir in the blueberries.

3 Spoon the mixture into the paper cases. Bake for 18–20 minutes until golden and well risen. Allow to cool for 5 minutes in the tin, then cool on a wire rack. These will keep for 3 days in an airtight container.

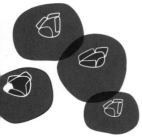

nutritional benefits
- *Provides vitamin A, vitamin C, calcium*

apricot, apple & oat cookies

Porridge is a morning staple, but there are so many other ways to make use of power-packed oats, including these cookies. Dried apricots are full of iron and vitamins A and C and provide a natural sweetness.

makes:
16 balls

1 apple peeled and grated
150g porridge oats
70g desiccated coconut
75g unsalted butter, melted
85ml maple syrup

1 tsp pure vanilla extract
1 egg
85g dried apricots, chopped
50g dates, chopped
1 tbsp chia seeds

1. Preheat the oven to 200°C (fan 180°C/gas mark 6). Line a baking tray with baking parchment.

2. Put the apple, oats, coconut, butter, maple syrup, vanilla and egg into a food processor. Whiz until roughly chopped.

3. Add the apricots, dates and seeds. Pulse again until combined. Shape into sixteen flat cookies.

4. Place on the lined tray and bake for 10–12 minutes until pale golden, turning over halfway through. Cool on a wire rack. These will keep in a tin for up to 5 days.

nutritional benefits
- *Nutritionally complete*
- *Provides vitamin C, iron (combination increases the absorption of iron)*
- *Source of prebiotics*

beetroot energy balls

Babies grow more rapidly in their first year than any other in their life and these balls will help to fuel their development and adventures!

makes:
30 balls

100g cooked beetroot, chopped
100g porridge oats
100g soft dates
100g smooth peanut butter
15g cocoa powder

2 tbsp maple syrup (*optional*)
1 tsp pure vanilla extract
50g pecans
50g desiccated coconut

1. Put all of the ingredients, except the coconut, into a food processor. Add 3 tablespoons of water and whiz until finely chopped.

2. Shape the mixture into thirty balls. Place the coconut in a bowl. Roll each ball in coconut. Chill for 30 minutes in the fridge. They will keep in an airtight container for up to 1 week.

nutritional benefits
- *Nutritionally complete*
- *Provides vitamin C and iron (combination increases the absorption of iron)*
- *Source of prebiotics*

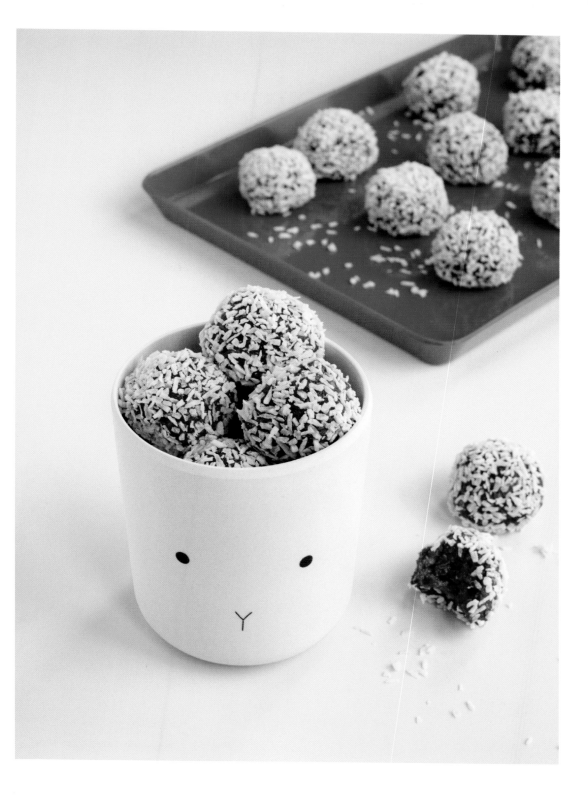

easy banana ice cream

I love to experiment in my kitchen and this two-ingredient recipe makes for the smoothest, creamiest ice cream. There is no cream, milk, eggs or sugar involved!

makes:
4 child portions

3 ripe bananas
1 tbsp smooth peanut butter

1. Peel the bananas and slice into rounds. Place on a baking tray lined with baking parchment, then put into the freezer for 2 hours.

2. Put the frozen banana slices into a food processor. Whiz on the pulse setting until finely chopped, then blend continually until it forms a smooth, thick ice cream texture. Add the peanut butter and whiz again until combined. You can eat it straight away or spoon into a container and freeze until needed.

nutritional benefits
- *Provides vitamin B6 and iron*

apple, oat & date balls

These mini balls are ideal for a snack on the go and will also still set your baby up for the day ahead as a breakfast.

makes:
20 balls

100g dates, chopped
1 eating apple, peeled and grated
½ tsp mixed spice
2 tbsp sunflower oil
1 tbsp maple syrup
100g oats

20g raisins
20g cranberries
1 tbsp flaxseeds
20g Rice Krispies
15g desiccated coconut

1. Put the dates and 75ml of cold water into a pan. Cover with a lid. Bring to the boil and boil for 5 minutes. Pour into a food processor.

2. Add the apple, mixed spice, oil and maple syrup and whiz until smooth. Add all the remaining ingredients apart from the desiccated coconut and whiz until roughly chopped. Shape the mixture into twenty balls.

3. Place the coconut in a bowl. Roll the balls in the coconut, to coat. Chill for 20 minutes in the fridge. They will keep in an airtight container for up to 1 week.

nutritional benefits
- *Nutritionally complete*
- *Provides omega 3s, vitamin C and iron
  (combination increases the absorption of iron)*
- *Source of prebiotics*

carrot, courgette & sweetcorn muffins

Introducing my nutritious savoury muffins with a trio of veggies. Full of flavour and ideal for fussy eaters, little ones will love pulling these apart and munching away.

makes:
12 muffins

You will also need
12-hole muffin tin
and muffin cases

280g self-raising flour
2 tsp baking powder
3 eggs
175ml milk
65g unsalted butter, melted
100g Parmesan cheese, grated

150g courgette, grated
75g carrot, peeled and grated
4 tbsp tinned sweetcorn
2 spring onions, sliced
1 tbsp chopped fresh thyme

1. Preheat the oven to 200°C (fan 180°C/gas mark 6). Line muffin tin with the paper cases.

2. Place the flour, baking powder and eggs into a mixing bowl. Add the milk and butter. Whisk until smooth. Fold in 80g of the Parmesan cheese and the remaining ingredients, mix well.

3. Spoon the mixture into the muffin cases and sprinkle with the remaining cheese. Bake for 25–30 minutes until well risen and golden brown. Leave to cool on a wire rack. They will keep in a tin for up to 1 week.

nutritional benefits
- *Nutritionally complete*
- *Provides vitamin D, vitamin E, vitamin C, iron (combination increases the absorption of iron) and calcium*
- *Source of prebiotics*

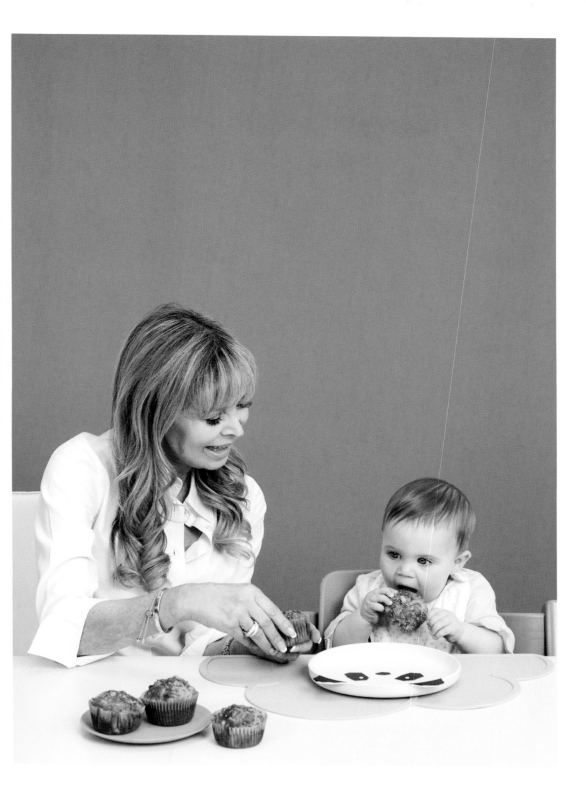

carrot cake energy balls

Power your baby's day with my healthy take on this
sweet treat.

makes:
30 balls

110g pecans
125g dates
200g carrots, peeled and grated
80g desiccated coconut
¾ tsp ground cinnamon

¾ tsp ground ginger
100g raisins
50g porridge oats
2 tbsp sunflower oil

1. Place all the ingredients into a food processor. Whiz until finely
    chopped.

2. Shape the mixture into thirty balls. Chill for 1 hour in the fridge.
    Keep in an airtight container in the fridge for up to 5 days.

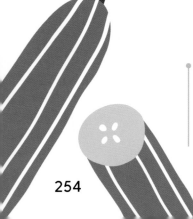

nutritional benefits
- *Nutritionally complete*
- *Provides vitamin C and iron (combination
  increases the absorption of iron)*
- *Source of prebiotics*

sushi sandwiches

Step-up your sandwich game and add a little theatre to the table with my sushi rolls. Move over sorry looking sandwiches, there's a new sarnie kid in the house!

makes:
12 pieces

2 eggs
2 tbsp shop-bought mayonnaise
2 slices of white bread
2 slices of brown bread
1 tomato, deseeded and diced

½ punnet cress
unsalted butter, for spreading
40g Cheddar cheese, grated
½ cucumber, sliced into thin
   batons

1. Put the eggs into a pan of cold water. Bring the water to the boil and boil the eggs for 10 minutes. Run under a cold tap and leave to cool, then peel and dice.

2. Mix the diced egg with the mayonnaise.

3. Remove the crusts from the bread. Roll out thinly using a rolling pin.

4. Spread the egg mayonnaise over the white bread. Sprinkle with tomato and cress. Roll up like a pinwheel. Slice into three pieces.

5. Spread a little butter over the brown bread. Top with Cheddar cheese and cucumber. Roll up like a pinwheel. Slice into three pieces.

nutritional benefits
- *Nutritionally complete*
- *Provides vitamin D, vitamin E, vitamin C, iron (combination increases the absorption of iron) and calcium*

WEEK 1

first tastes meal planners
FROM AROUND 6 MONTHS

The **FIRST TASTES MEAL PLANNER: WEEK 1** is suitable for both a spoon-led or baby-led weaning approach. If you are going down the baby-led route, with baby taking the lead, then instead of puréeing you will need to steam the vegetables or offer wedges of no-cook fruit so that they are nice and soft for your baby to hold. In addition to the milk feeds shown in the table, your baby may also need a mid-afternoon and night-time feed.

If weaning occurs at 6 months, be aware that your baby's nutritional needs for certain key nutrients such as iron are not met by milk alone. They will therefore need to quite quickly progress to foods that are rich in these nutrients (see page 44 for more information) to ensure they are getting the correct amount of critical nutrients in their diet such as iron and essential fatty acids.

DAY	EARLY MORNING	BREAKFAST	LUNCH	TEA	BEDTIME
1	Breast / Bottle	Breast / Bottle	Vegetable purée eg. carrot / sweet potato	Breast / Bottle	Breast / Bottle
2	Breast / Bottle	Breast / Bottle	Mashed avocado	Breast / Bottle	Breast / Bottle
3	Breast / Bottle	Breast / Bottle	Apple purée	Breast / Bottle	Breast / Bottle
4	Breast / Bottle	Breast / Bottle	Carrot **or** butternut squash purée	Breast / Bottle	Breast / Bottle
5	Breast / Bottle	Breast / Bottle	Broccoli purée	Breast / Bottle	Breast / Bottle
6	Breast / Bottle	Breast / Bottle	Carrot **or** butternut squash purée	Breast / Bottle	Breast / Bottle
7	Breast / Bottle	Breast / Bottle	Mashed banana	Breast / Bottle	Breast / Bottle

FIRST TASTES & COMBINED PURÉES

Here are some suggestions of first tastes fruit and vegetables for your baby to enjoy at the beginning of her weaning journey.

Start with the main ingredient in the column on the left. The reason for this is so that your baby can identify the foods she is eating. When she has accepted these single flavours, then add one, two or three ingredients from the other columns. Mix and match to find out your baby's favourite flavour combinations!

Carrot	Sweet potato Parsnip Butternut squash Cauliflower Sweet pepper Potato	Parsnip Apple Cauliflower Spinach Sweetcorn Butternut squash Broccoli
Sweet Potato	Potato Butternut squash Red pepper Pea Carrot	Pea Broccoli Cauliflower Spinach Leek Parsnip Cauliflower
Apple	Pear Blueberry Pear Strawberry Peach Prune	Banana Prune Banana Strawberry
Banana	Avocado Mango Apple Peach Strawberry Prune	Dried apricot Blueberry Mango Full-fat yoghurt

WEEKS 2 & 3

The **AFTER FIRST TASTES MEAL PLANNER: WEEKS 2–3** takes you through to introducing varied foods after first tastes when your baby is ready for more.

Every baby is different and will develop at her own pace. So, let her guide you towards when she might be ready to move on to two meals a day. You can be flexible – it's about making it work for you. For example, it might be that breakfast and tea works better for you and your family's routine. The same applies with your baby's milk feeds. As a guide, your baby will be having roughly four milk feeds a day – but feel free to interchange the milk feed that is offered alongside their meal.

DAY	EARLY MORNING	BREAKFAST	LUNCH	TEA	BEDTIME
1	Breast / Bottle	Apple & pear purée **or** steamed apple wedges & fresh pear Breast / Bottle	Sweet potato & spinach purée **or** sweet potato batons	Breast / Bottle	Breast / Bottle
2	Breast / Bottle	Avocado & banana purée **or** finger food Breast / Bottle	Carrot & parsnip purée **or** carrot and parsnip batons	Breast / Bottle	Breast / Bottle
3	Breast / Bottle	Mango & banana purée **or** finger food Breast / Bottle	Baked butternut squash & roasted sweet pepper purée **or** finger food	Breast / Bottle	Breast / Bottle
4	Breast / Bottle	Apple purée & iron-fortified baby cereal **or** finger food Breast / Bottle	Sweet potato & spinach purée **or** finger food	Breast / Bottle	Breast / Bottle
5	Breast / Bottle	Peach or mango & banana purée **or** finger food Breast / Bottle	Parsnip & apple purée **or** finger food	Breast / Bottle	Breast / Bottle
6	Breast / Bottle	Apple & pear with iron-fortified baby cereal **or** finger food Breast / Bottle	Baked butternut squash & broccoli purée **or** finger food	Breast / Bottle	Breast / Bottle
7	Breast / Bottle	Banana & blueberry purée **or** finger food Breast / Bottle	Carrot & parsnip purée **or** batons	Breast / Bottle	Breast / Bottle

WEEK 4

The **AFTER FIRST TASTES MEAL PLANNER: WEEK 4** introduces protein and more varied foods. Mealtimes can be interchangeable and the same applies for milk feeds too. For example, you might want to offer your baby her usual milk feed alongside breakfast (as opposed to tea as per the below).

DAY	EARLY MORNING	BREAKFAST	LUNCH	TEA	BEDTIME
1	Breast / Bottle	Banana & blueberry purée **or** chunks of banana and fresh blueberries	Breast / Bottle	Chicken, quinoa, apple & sage balls **or** purée (page 136) Breast / Bottle	Breast /Bottle
2	Breast / Bottle	Apple & strawberry with iron-rich cereal	Breast / Bottle	Salmon, sweet potato & spinach purée (page 120) **or** cooked flaked salmon and batons of sweet potato Breast / Bottle	Breast /Bottle
3	Breast / Bottle	Yoghurt, banana & prune purée (page 93)	Breast / Bottle	Beef, carrot & sweet potato purée (page 151) **or** Mini meatballs with carrot & apple (page 152) Breast/ Bottle	Breast /Bottle
4	Breast / Bottle	Scrambled egg & toast fingers	Breast / Bottle	Lentil & sweet potato bites **or** purée (page 114) Breast / Bottle	Breast /Bottle
5	Breast / Bottle	Porridge with blueberry, pear & apple (page 96)	Breast / Bottle	Chicken, quinoa, apple & sage balls **or** purée (page 136) Breast / Bottle	Breast / Bottle
6	Breast / Bottle	Toast fingers with peanut butter **or** cream cheese and fruit	Breast / Bottle	Lentil, kale & carrot purée (page 114) **or** flaked cooked salmon and sweet potato batons Breast / Bottle	Breast / Bottle
7	Breast / Bottle	Apple & strawberry with iron-fortified baby cereal	Breast / Bottle	Salmon, sweet potato & spinach purée (page 120) **or** flaked cooked salmon and sweet potato batons Breast / Bottle	Breast / Bottle

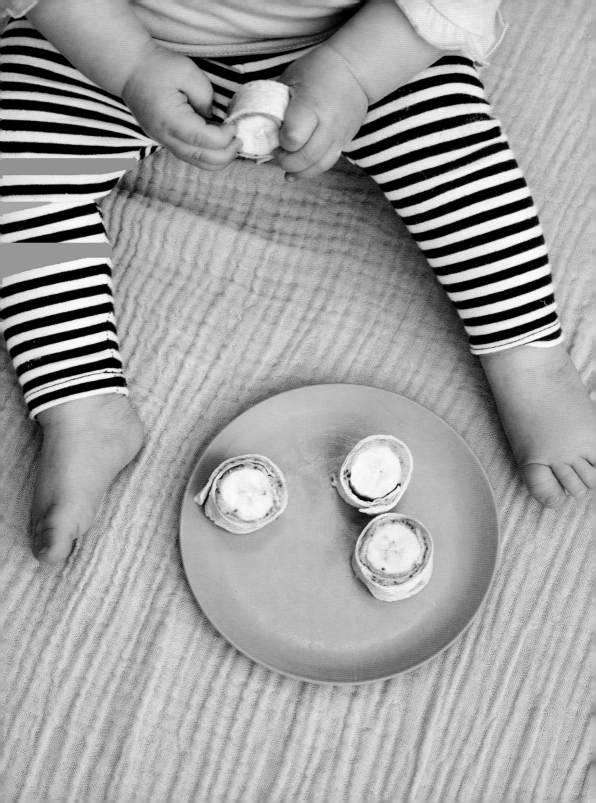

second stage meal planners
6–9 MONTHS

The **SECOND STAGE MEAL PLANNER** is for when your baby has progressed to eating three meals a day (see meal planners from pages 258–260 to show how to do this). She may be 6 or 7 months old by this point. As well as the milk feeds on this planner, your baby may need a mid-morning and night-time feed. Don't forget that with all of my meal planners, it is absolutely fine to repeat recipes. Plus, after all, most of the recipes make multiple portions and can be frozen too!

	BREAKFAST	LUNCH	MID AFTERNOON	TEA	BEDTIME
1	Yoghurt, banana & prune purée (page 93)	Chicken with apricots (page 132)	Breast / Bottle	Beef, carrot & sweet potato purée (page 151)	Breast / Bottle
2	Scrambled egg with spinach & tomatoes (page 96)	Salmon & sweet potato croquettes (page 124)	Breast / Bottle	Tomato and butternut squash pasta (page 110)	Breast / Bottle
3	Weetabix with apple purée (page 93)	Chicken, quinoa, apple & sage balls **or** purée (page 136)	Breast / Bottle	Roasted sweet potato wedges Fruit	Breast / Bottle
4	Porridge with blueberry, pear & apple (page 96)	Lentil & sweet potato bites **or** purée (page 114)	Breast / Bottle	Mini meatballs with carrot & apple (page 152)	Breast / Bottle
5	Toast fingers with peanut butter **or** cream cheese & fruit	Courgette & broccoli frittata (page 108)	Breast / Bottle	Salmon in tomato sauce with baby pasta shells (page 122)	Breast / Bottle
6	Iron-fortified baby cereal & berries	Quinoa with Mediterranean vegetables (page 112)	Breast / Bottle	Cod, spinach, potato & pea purée (page 126)	Breast / Bottle
7	Cheese & chive omelette (page 95)	Mini meatballs with carrot & apple (page 152)	Breast / Bottle	Tomato & butternut squash pasta (page 110)	Breast / Bottle

VEGETARIAN 6–9 MONTHS PLANNER

If you are weaning your baby on a vegetarian diet, then from 6 months it's important to be extra careful you make up for any shortfalls in their diet to ensure they are getting the critical nutrients (in particular iron and B12) for their long-term health and development.

As well as the milk feeds shown in the table below, your baby may also need a mid-morning and night-time feed. Some of these meals are not marked as vegetarian in the book because they include Parmesan — you can use vegetarian hard cheese if you prefer.

DAY	BREAKFAST	LUNCH	MID AFTERNOON	TEA	BEDTIME
1	Yoghurt, banana & prune purée (page 93)	Lentil & sweet potato bites **or** purée (page 114)	Breast / Bottle	Spinach pasta with butternut squash (page 106)	Breast / Bottle
2	Scrambled egg with spinach & tomatoes (page 96)	Roasted vegetables (page 103)	Breast / Bottle	Carrot, sweet potato & lentils with Pasta (page 111)	Breast / Bottle
3	Yoghurt pancakes with berries (page 158)	Quinoa with Mediterranean vegetables (page 112)	Breast / Bottle	Butternut squash & broccoli purée (page 105)	Breast / Bottle
4	Porridge with blueberry, pear & apple (page 96)	Lentil & sweet potato bites **or** purée (page 114)	Breast / Bottle	Tomato & butternut squash pasta (page 110))	Breast / Bottle
5	Toast fingers with peanut butter & fruit	Courgette & broccoli frittata (page 108)	Breast / Bottle	Quinoa with Mediterranean vegetables (page 112)	Breast / Bottle
6	Iron-fortified cereal & berries	Tomato & butternut squash pasta (page 110)	Breast / Bottle	Courgette & broccoli frittata (page 108)	Breast / Bottle
7	Yoghurt pancakes with berries (page 158)	Broccoli, sweet potato & chickpea croquettes (p 00)	Breast / Bottle	Spinach pasta with butternut squash (page 106)	Breast / Bottle

growing independence meal planner
9–12 MONTHS

Your baby will be exploring flavours and sampling small portions of family meals. From around 9–10 months she may have a small mid-morning or afternoon snack instead of milk feeds, and have a morning and evening milk feed as well as a smaller one during the day. Babies typically need two milk feeds with calcium-rich yoghurt or cheese per day, or three milk feeds. Milk feeds and snacking differs for babies, so that's why the meal planner is flexible accordingly. Feel free to repeat recipes, ensuring that she has two portions of oily fish a week and plenty of iron-rich recipes every day.

DAY	AM	BREAKFAST	MID AM	LUNCH	MID PM	TEA	BEDTIME
1	Breast / Bottle	Baby muesli & berries	Snack or Breast / Bottle	Mini Cottage Pies (page 228) Fruit	Snack or Breast / Bottle	Salmon with pasta shells (page 208) Carrot cake energy balls (page 254)	Breast / Bottle
2	Breast / Bottle	Scrambled egg with spinach & tomatoes (page 96) Fruit	Snack or Breast / Bottle	Herby chicken goujons with tomato & basil sauce with broccoli (page 220)	Snack or Breast / Bottle	Frittata muffins (page 190) Yoghurt	Breast / Bottle
3	Breast / Bottle	Banana eggy bread (page 165) Fruit	Snack or Breast / Bottle	Haddock, potato & sweetcorn chowder (page 205) Beetroot, strawberry & blueberry lolly (page 174)	Snack or Breast / Bottle	Roast chicken with sweet potato, thyme and peppers (page 212) Fruit	Breast / Bottle
4	Breast / Bottle	Soft boiled egg with Welsh rarebit toast (page 164) Fruit	Snack or Breast / Bottle	Carrot cake energy balls (page 254) Butternut squash, red onion and pepper meatballs (page 230) Squash wedges	Snack or Breast / Bottle	Yogurt-based pizza margherita (page 236) Easy banana ice cream (page 250)	Breast / Bottle
5	Breast / Bottle	Overnight oats with berries & seeds (page 166) Yogurt	Snack or Breast / Bottle	Scrummy salmon noodles with veggies (page 197) Beetroot, strawberry & blueberry lolly (page 174)	Snack or Breast / Bottle	Cauliflower, couscous, kale and lentils (page 194) Fruit	Breast / Bottle
6	Breast / Bottle	Yoghurt, banana & seed loaf (page 162) Fruit	Snack or Breast / Bottle	Bolognese pasta bake (page 232) Peach & raspberry yoghurt pot (page 247)	Snack or Breast / Bottle	Lentil, sweet potato & kale with tomatoes (page 185) Yoghurt	Breast / Bottle
7	Breast / Bottle	Baby muesli & berries	Snack or Breast / Bottle	Curried chicken and veggie croquettes (page 217) Fruit	Snack or Breast / Bottle	Tuna pasta bake (page 206) Easy banana ice cream (page 252)	Breast / Bottle

index

Page numbers in **bold** refer to images

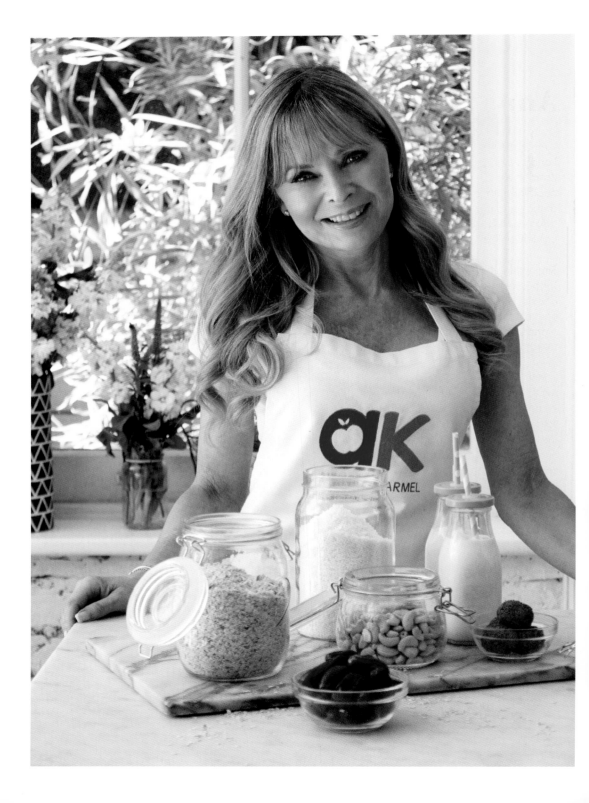

Annabel Karmel MBE

With expertise spanning more than 27 years, London-born mother of three Annabel Karmel reigns as the UK's no. 1 children's cookery author, bestselling international author, and a world-leading expert on devising delicious, nutritious meals for babies, children and families.

Since launching her revolutionary cookbook for babies in 1991 – a feeding 'bible', which has become the 2nd bestselling non-fiction hardback of all time – Annabel has pioneered the way families all over the world feed their babies and children.

A leading expert and entrepreneur within the food industry, Annabel has cooked-up 46 books, with more than 6 million copies sold globally. Her menus can also be found in the world's largest hotels and leisure resorts and her expert range of award-winning children's meals can be found in major UK and international supermarkets including Australia, Europe and China. Nutritionally balanced and inspired by her homemade recipes, Annabel's chilled and frozen meals have become a trusted solution for those busy days.

With millions of families relying on Annabel's recipes to raise healthy, happy babies, it is no surprise that Annabel has a phenomenal digital and social following, coupled with a no. 1 ranking recipe app. Packed with over 350 delicious, nutritious recipes, simple planners, shopping lists and more, it's the handiest of guides for easy mealtime inspiration –whether you're cooking for baby, toddler or the whole family.

From kitchen table to global stage, Annabel uses her revolutionary food platform to campaign for better food standards, raise essential funds for charity, support women in business and share advice at business and entrepreneurial forums. In 2006, Annabel received an MBE in the Queen's Birthday Honours for her outstanding work in the field of child nutrition, and she is also well recognised as one of the UK's leading female entrepreneurs.

For lots more exclusive recipes, tips and advice, plus a host of great competitions and offers, join the AK Club for free today at **www.annabelkarmel.com**. You can also be a part of Annabel's world on social media.

@annabelkarmeluk
@annabelkarmel

with thanks

Writing a book is like having a baby! It's a lot of fun at the beginning trying out lots of different concepts, then generally 9 months gestation and a flurry of activity with a certain amount of pain at the end to get everything 'delivered'. I am super fussy when it comes to food which means that only the very best tried-and-tested recipes that get the thumbs up and clean plates make it into the book. I couldn't do this without the wonderful team at Bluebird and at AK HQ plus the tremendous patience of my family and friends and tiny tasters.

Thank you to Carole Tonkinson, Lucinda McCord, Lucy Staley, Jonathan Lloyd, Martha Burley, Sarah Smith, Ellis Parrinder, Lara Karmel, Scarlett Karmel, Nick Karmel, Evelyn Etkind, Stephen Margolis, Marina Abaigon Magpoc, Charlie Phillips, Nikki Dupin, Lizzie Harris, Jenny Estacio and Robyn Colton.

Thanks to JoJo Maman Bébé for loaning the baby clothes for the shoot.

the models

With thanks to our wonderful models:

Emilia Ivy Dickinson
Camille Echaubard
Mia Kilby
Suri Metha
Arnie Beck Patel
Cairo-Soul Antionette D'nai Powell-Ankers
Elliot John Wake

About Rosan Meyer M. Nutr, PhD

Rosan Meyer is a dietitian who finished her specialisation in paediatrics in 2000. She then went on to do a MSc in Paediatric Nutrition and completed her PhD at Imperial College London in 2008. She has worked in well-known paediatric tertiary hospitals. She currently has a private paediatric dietetic practice specialising in food allergy, feeding difficulties and faltering growth in London. In addition, she is honorary senior lecturer at Imperial College, London UK and visiting Professor at KU Leuven, Belgium. She is the author of more than 50 peer-reviewed articles on paediatric nutrition and book chapters, and serves on many national and international associations involved in paediatric nutrition.